D1823200

Proceedings of the Symposium on
EPIDURAL ANALGESIA
IN OBSTETRICS

Kingston Hospital, Kingston-upon-Thames, 18th March 1971

Editor: ANDREW DOUGHTY, MB, BS, FFARCS

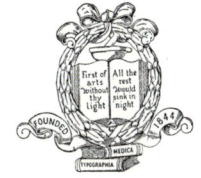

LONDON
H. K. LEWIS & Co. Ltd.
1972

BDH PHARMACEUTICALS LIMITED LONDON E2

©

BDH PHARMACEUTICALS LTD
1972

STANDARD BOOK NO
0 7186 0382 6

Printed in England by
ASHMEAD PRESS LTD
LONDON SE10

Foreword

This is the report of a Symposium which, it was felt by many among those who attended, was particularly lively and of absorbing interest. During the course of the day's activities it became quite plain that the seal was being set upon the establishment of a new phase in British obstetric practice. For a quarter of a century after the introduction by Hingson of the concept of continuous epidural block to relieve the pain of labour and delivery, only a few isolated enthusiasts among the anaesthetists and obstetricians of this country could be found to apply the technique. This long latent period resulted from several factors: in part it was due to a relative shortage of anaesthetists, in part it reflected the general lack of concern shown by British anaesthetists in obstetric matters, and a contributory factor was doubtless the considerable frequency with which topping-up doses were required when using the drugs then available. However, beneath the surface of events, a quiet evolution was continuing, and it required only the appropriate catalyst to turn the quantitative change into a qualitative one. The catalyst proved to be the Fourth World Congress of Anaesthesiologists, held in 1968 in London. The reporting of discussions about the use of epidural block in obstetrics in the press and on television and radio aroused much public interest which provided the spur to many anaesthetists and obstetricians. The vast surge of interest and application persists, and it might be said that this Symposium represents the point of no return. It is now generally acknowledged that the provision of epidural analgesia in labour, for all except those in whom it is contra-indicated, is a practical proposition, and that this form of pain relief is outstandingly the most efficient yet devised.

What has permitted this dramatic burgeoning of 'epidural services'? Firstly, in recent years, there has been a most welcome appreciation of the challenge and interest of obstetric problems in relation to anaesthesia. This resulted in the formation, in 1969, of the Obstetric Anaesthetists' Association (O.A.A.), an organisation primarily concerned with raising the standards of patient care in obstetrics with respect to anaesthesia, analgesia and neonatal resuscitation. The Association is composed mainly of consultant anaesthetists whose daily work presents them with problems in these areas. One of the main matters of immediate concern to the O.A.A. has been the tragically high incidence of maternal deaths associated with anaesthesia in this country; another has been the evolution of a widespread and safe practice of lumbar epidural analgesia for labour and delivery. The Symposium reported here was held under the auspices of the O.A.A., and one fact which passed almost unremarked at the meeting itself, but is striking in retrospect, is not so much the high quality of the contributions but from whence they came. Well-known figures from the national and international circuits were not flown in to present the tablets from on high and then depart. This was a Symposium of working people describing their own observations made in the context of clinical experience, and the many and informed discussants from the body of the hall were similarly reflecting difficulties and successes which they had personally experienced. It was this maintained tenor of involved interest which distinguished the Symposium in the manner which I have described. I

3

hope, and believe, that at least some of that interest will be discerned by the readers of this book.

There seems little reason for doubting that lumbar epidural analgesia will, during the coming years, provide complete relief from pain in labour for increasing numbers of women in this country. If it is not indeed a fact now, certainly within five years there will be more lumbar epidural blocks given in the United Kingdom each year than in any other country, which is as it should be, as we have incomparably the largest number per capita of competent and experienced anaesthetists. Within the next few years bupivacaine, which has taken so much of the toil from 'topping up', may have been superseded, pain in labour will be an uncommon event, and the O.A.A. will be concerning itself with matters other than the setting up of epidural services. It will, I am sure, have initiated many other Symposia of equal importance and interest. However, I believe that this Symposium will still be recalled as a landmark of some note in the history of both anaesthesia and obstetrics in this country. It is fitting therefore, that tribute finally be paid to the members of the Department of Anaesthetics, Kingston Hospital, who have worked indefatigably to organise and to sustain the Symposium and to gather the material from often slothful contributors to fashion it, within a remarkably short time, into the present volume.

J. SELWYN CRAWFORD
Convener
Obstetric Anaesthetists' Association

Preface

Under the auspices of the Obstetric Anaesthetists' Association a Symposium on Epidural Analgesia in Labour was held at Kingston Hospital on March 18th, 1971. The event attracted 160 anaesthetists and obstetricians and included representatives from nearly all the centres in Great Britain and Northern Ireland where the technique is practised. The programme included contributions on most facets of the subject. The time allocated to invited speakers was strictly limited so as to give ample opportunity for discussion from the floor. While there was a wide range of opinion expressed, there was a common theme of concern for the welfare of both mother and baby.

A general welcome for epidural analgesia was tempered by the conviction that freedom from trouble could only be achieved by skill, experience and meticulous attention to detail. Many papers drew attention to the pressing need for more original research into the many aspects of a comparatively neglected field of modern anaesthetic practice. This publication is an edited recording of the proceedings and is offered as a cross-section of current opinion on epidural analgesia in the United Kingdom in 1971.

ANDREW DOUGHTY
Editor

Acknowledgments

To Mrs. Helen Ferrelly and Mrs. Norah Wilmot, secretaries to the Department of Anaesthetics, Kingston Hospital, has fallen the formidable task of organising the Symposium, transcribing the proceedings, corresponding with participants and typing the various versions of the manuscript. The Convener and members of the Committee of the Obstetric Anaesthetists' Association would like to thank them for their invaluable assistance. They would also like to record their appreciation of the generosity of BDH Pharmaceuticals Limited for support of the Symposium and for meeting the cost of the publication of the proceedings. A tribute is due in particular to Mr. P. A. Langley, their Publicity Manager, without whose constant help this booklet would never have been published.

List of Participants

Chairman of Symposium: ANDREW DOUGHTY, MB, BS, FFARCS,
Kingston Hospital,
Kingston-upon-Thames, Surrey.

Participants:

R ARMSTRONG, MB, BCh, BAO, FFARCS,
Ulster Hospital,
Dundonald, Co. Down.

R S ATKINSON, MB, BChir, FFARCS,
Southend-on-Sea Hospital,
Essex.

T H L BRYSON, MB, ChB, FFARCS,
United Liverpool Hospitals.

J M B BURN, MB, ChB, FFARCS, DObstRCOG,
Southampton General Hospital.

L E S CARRIE, MB, ChB, FFARCS,
United Oxford Hospitals.

B CHATTERJEE, MB, BS, MRCOG,
Sorrento Maternity Hospital,
Birmingham.

R J H COLBACK, MB, ChB, FFARCS, DTM & H,
Newcastle General Hospital,
Newcastle-upon-Tyne.

KENNETH COOPER, MB, BS, FRCSEd, MRCOG,
Worthing Hospital Group,
Sussex.

J SELWYN CRAWFORD, MB, ChB, FFARCS,
Birmingham Maternity Hospital.

I T DAVIE, MB, ChB, FFARCS,
Royal Infirmary,
Edinburgh.

C J MASSEY DAWKINS, MA, MD, FFARCS,
University College Hospital,
London, WC 1.

O P DINNICK, MB, BS, FFARCS,
Middlesex Hospital,
London, W 1.

J F EDMONDS, MB, BS, FFARCS,
University College Hospital,
London, WC 1.

J FRAMPTON, MD, MRCOG,
South Warwickshire Hospital Group.

J FRASER JONES, MB, BS, FFARCS,
Solihull and East Birmingham Hospitals.

RONALD GREEN, MA, MB, BChir, FFARCS,
St George's and Royal Free Hospitals,
London.

R L HARGROVE, MB, BS, FFARCS,
Westminster Hospital,
London, SW 1.

D C HUGHES, MB, BS, FFARCS,
St Peter's Hospital,
Chertsey, Surrey.

DONALD D MOIR, MD, FFARCS, DObstRCOG,
Queen Mother's Hospital,
Glasgow.

A D G NICHOLAS, MB, BChir, FFARCS,
United Sheffield Hospitals.

A D NOBLE, MB, BS, FRCSEd, MRCOG, DCH,
Westminster Hospital,
London, SW 1.

J F PEARSON, MB, BS, MRCOG,
Birmingham Maternity Hospital.

J E REDMEN, MD, BPharm, FFARCS,
Guildford & Godalming Group,
Surrey.

FELICITY REYNOLDS, MB, BS, FFARCS,
St Thomas's Hospital,
London, SE 1.

M ROSEN, MB, ChB, FFARCS,
United Cardiff Hospitals.

A P RUBIN, MB, BChir, FFARCS,
Charing Cross Hospital,
London, WC 2.

D B SCOTT, MD, FFARCS,
Royal Infirmary,
Edinburgh.

Prof. B R J SIMPSON, DPhil, FFARCS, DObstRCOG,
London Hospital,
London, E 1.

T R STEEN, MB, BChir, FFARCS,
Southmead Hospital,
Bristol.

M E TUNSTALL, MB, BS, FFARCS, DObstRCOG,
Royal Infirmary,
Aberdeen.

J WILSON, MB, ChB, FFARCS, DObstRCOG,
United Leeds Hospitals.

T M YOUNG, MB, BS, FFARCS,
United Manchester Hospitals.

SYMPOSIUM
on
EPIDURAL ANALGESIA IN OBSTETRICS
Chairman—DR ANDREW DOUGHTY

Epidural Analgesia and Pain Pathways in Labour

DR ANDREW DOUGHTY (Kingston-upon-Thames)

In 1969 Professor Jeffcoate, President of the Royal College of Obstetricians and Gynaecologists, admitted that he found difficulty in deciding to what extent anatomically demonstrable autonomic nerves carry impulses to and from the blood vessels and to what extent they are motor or sensory to other tissues. He added that it is not known whether the uterus receives both parasympathetic and sympathetic nerves or whether it receives only a sympathetic component.[1]

Patterns of Pain in Labour
Many of us take a somewhat empirical view of relieving labour pain by epidural analgesia. An injection of 7 ml bupivacaine in the mid-lumbar region will satisfy the majority of mothers and it is only when this fails to produce the desired effect that one begins to wonder what is amiss. It is therefore worth considering not only how one should relieve labour pain but also what pain one is actually trying to relieve.

Figure 1

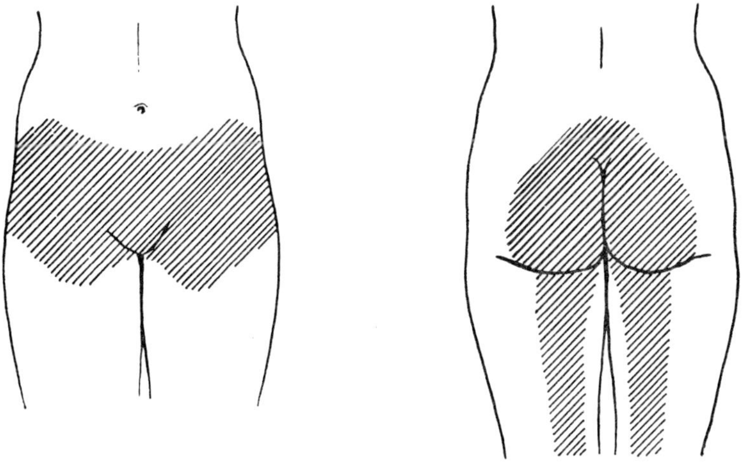

Cutaneous Distribution of Pain in Labour (Wylie 1953)

Figure 1 is taken from Wylie's 'Practical Management of Pain in Labour'[2] and suggests that women in labour experience pain either in the hypogastrium referable to the dermatomes supplied by T11, 12 and L.1 or in the back referable to the area supplied by S2, 3 and 4. It is rather an attractive proposition, of course, not borne out in practice, that if the mother feels pain in the front the block should be directed at the lower thoracic and upper lumbar segments and that if she feels pain over the sacrum the block should affect the 2nd, 3rd and 4th sacral roots. Nevertheless back pain associated with the uterine contractions can usually be

9

relieved by a small-volume epidural injection given at the T11-12 interspace. I have yet to see a satisfactory explanation for this paradox.

A discomfort of early labour is the backache which disappears when the head starts to descend into the pelvis. This is thought to be due to pressure of the foetal head on the anterior aspect of the sacrum and is presumably mediated by the somatic sacral roots.[3] Towards the end of the first stage there is the sensation of rectal pressure which may become so intolerable as to demand relief. In the second stage there is the discomfort, variable in intensity, of the stretching of the perineum which may not require specific relief as long as the pain of uterine contraction remains abolished. It is curious that many women under epidural analgesia seem to be able to tolerate the stretching and even the tearing of the perineum without a sign of discomfort, but complain of the pain of perineal suture immediately following parturition.

My personal records show that the pain of uterine contraction is felt in the hypogastrium by 70% and in the back by 20% of women. Having attended many individual mothers in successive labours, it appears that pain in the back is a personal characteristic and is not necessarily related to inco-ordinate uterine action or occipito-posterior position. The remaining 10% of mothers either complain of hypogastric and sacral pain of equal intensity or of more unusual pain patterns. For instance unilateral or bilateral *sciatic* pain was the only complaint in some labours, and in others the main cause of distress was severe pain limited to the iliac fossa on one side only. To complete the picture of unusual patterns of labour there were a few mothers who denied any discomfort whatever throughout the whole course of labour.

Figure 2

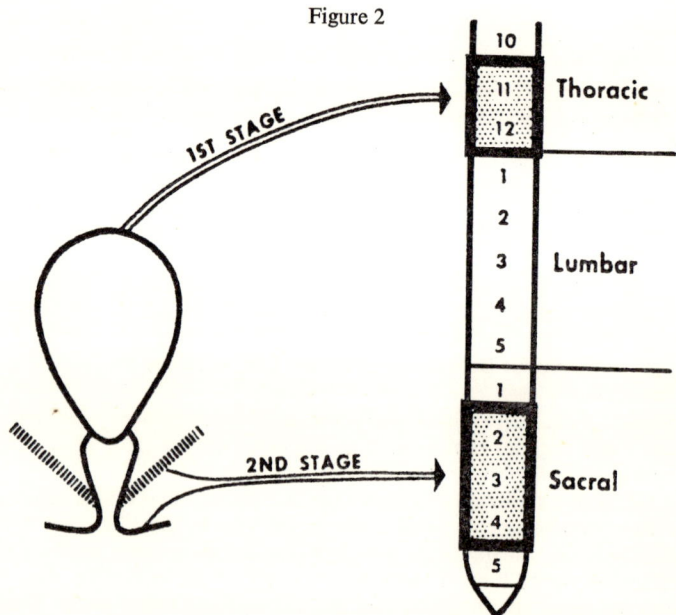

Dual Pathways of Pain in Labour (Bromage 1961)

Relief of Pain by Epidural Block

Figure 2 is taken from a paper by Bromage[4] and shows the dual pathways of pain impulses from the genital tract to the central nervous system. It suggests that the pain of the first stage of labour is relieved by blockade of the lower two thoracic segments and that of the second stage by blockade of the sacral segments. The uninitiated might interpret this diagram as suggesting that at full dilatation of the cervix the sacral segments take over the function of transmission of labour pain and that a saddle or pudendal nerve block would provide complete relief. Nothing is further from the truth. Sacral block provides analgesia of the pelvic floor and suitable conditions for forceps delivery. The pain of uterine contractions continues throughout labour and its relief demands blockade of the lower thoracic segments in both the first and second stages. Conversely an epidural block affecting only the lower thoracic segments at or near full dilatation of the cervix may give incomplete relief of maternal distress and a block of the sacral roots may be necessary in addition. A not uncommon situation occurs when the primary epidural block is given supposedly at about 4-5 cm dilatation of the cervix for severe hypogastric or sacral pain. Unexpectedly the mother remains distressed although she admits that the pain of which she originally complained has been alleviated. The complaint is now of intolerable pressure on the rectum or pelvic floor. Examination reveals that she has unexpectedly progressed to the second stage; blockade of the sacral roots restores her composure.

Figure 3

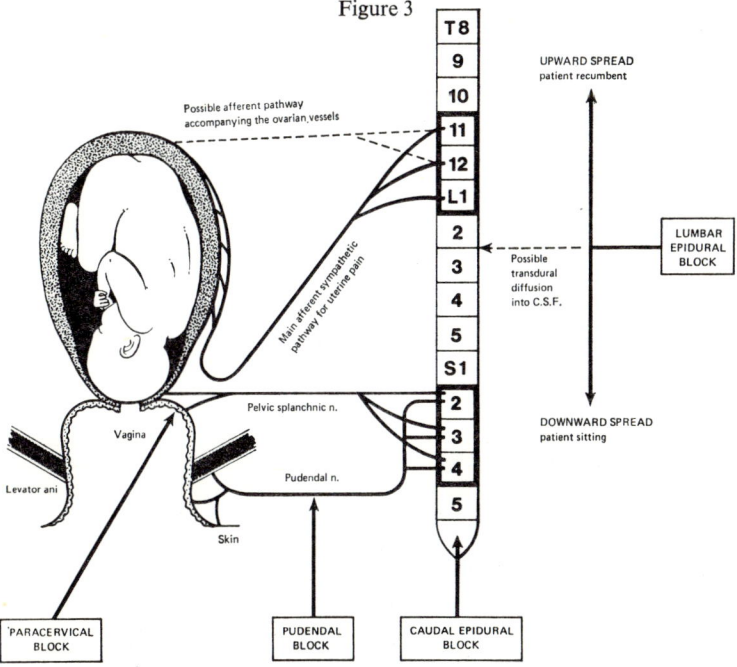

Pain Pathways in Labour in relation to Conduction Block (Wylie and Churchill-Davidson 1972)

Principles of Conduction Block in Labour

I must take some responsibility for Figure 3 which summarises the rationale of the various conduction blocks used in labour. The main afferent pathway for uterine pain passes from the uterus through the base of the broad ligament to the pelvic, hypogastric and aortico-renal plexuses to enter the central nervous system through the lower thoracic and upper lumbar segments. There may possibly be an afferent pathway accompanying the ovarian vessels through the infundibulo-pelvic ligament direct into the lower thoracic segments via the aortico-renal plexus. The pelvic splanchnic nerve has long been thought to transmit pain impulses from the cervix and upper vagina to the 2nd, 3rd and 4th sacral segments particularly the severe backache associated with inco-ordinate uterine action and occipito-posterior positions. Its inclusion in this diagram is more out of respect for tradition than on account of any convincing evidence of its function. The pudendal nerve transmits sensation from the lower vagina and pelvic floor and, in addition, supplies the musculature of that region.

Paracervical block should interrupt both the main afferent pathway and the pelvic splanchnic nerve. It cannot affect the possible alternative pathway from the fundus of the uterus accompanying the ovarian vessels[5], neither does it relieve the discomfort of pelvic floor pressure transmitted by the pudendal nerve. The sloping arrow suggests the direction in which the injection should be made to avoid the risk of penetrating the uterus and the intervillous space.

The limited field of the effect of pudendal nerve block when used for forceps delivery is a reminder that patients continue to feel the pain of labour despite the efficient performance of the block.

The diagram illustrates the distinction between caudal and lumbar epidural analgesia. An injection through the caudal canal primarily blocks the sacral roots usually long before there is any need to do so. Relatively large volumes of local anaesthetic solution must be injected in order to affect the lower thoracic segments. Smaller volumes will produce a saddle block without relieving labour pain. Successive top-ups reinforce the sacral blockade producing total relaxation of the pelvic floor, and instrumental delivery must be anticipated in most cases. A forceps rate of only 25% has been claimed when the more selective lumbar route is used[6].

With lumbar epidural block the injection is made nearer to the lower thoracic region, relatively smaller doses are required to relieve uterine pain and initially the sacral roots remain unaffected. It is usual to achieve relief of uterine pain by an injection of about 7 ml of local anaesthetic at the 2nd-3rd lumber interspace with the mother lying horizontally. If sacral block is required later in labour an injection of 8-10 ml is given through the catheter with the patient sitting up. There are those who place the initial injection at the 11th-12th thoracic interspace and effectively relieve uterine pain with as little as 3 ml of local anaesthetic solution. However there may be some difficulty in achieving a subsequent sacral block by injecting through the cannula at this relatively high level.

One fairly constant feature of lumbar epidural analgesia is that the majority of women deliver without complaint and without demanding any formal attempt to block the sacral roots. Either the stretching of the pelvic floor is relatively painless, particularly in multiparae, or the sacral roots are partially or completely blocked quite fortuitously without any specific attempts being made to do so. In many cases, after one or two top-ups, the perineum becomes numb without the patient having been placed in the sitting position. Yet uterine pain may return in the second stage of labour while the perineum remains anaesthetised. I do not know what is the explanation. Does the local anaesthetic spread downwards in the epidural space while waning in effect in the lower thoracic region, or is there a gradual diffusion directly across the dura into the cerebrospinal fluid [7] so that the cauda equina becomes blocked?

Occasionally an injection through the catheter in the lumbar region fails to achieve a sacral block despite the use of large volumes with the patient sitting up. One can only postulate some factor preventing the spread of local anaesthetic in the epidural space. The relief of perineal pain in late labour can then only be obtained by a supplementary pudendal, caudal or saddle subarachnoid block. These observations point to the deficiencies in our knowledge of the anatomy of the epidural space and of the spread of solutions injected into it.

As long as eminent authorities disclaim certainty as to the function of the afferent nerves serving the genital tract, it would be rash to suggest that Figure 3 illustrates the definite proved neural pathways of pain in labour. I can only offer it as a working hypothesis for the practice of epidural analgesia and, on the present occasion, as a basis for discussion.

REFERENCES

1. Jeffcoate T N A (1969). *Pelvic Pain*, Brit. med. J. **3,** 431
2. Wylie W D (1953). *The Practical Management of Pain in Labour*, Lloyd-Luke, London.
3. Crawford J S (1965). *Principles and Practice of Obstetric Anaesthesia*, 2nd Edition, p.25 Blackwell, Oxford
4. Bromage P R (1961). *Continuous Lumbar Epidural Analgesia for Obstetrics.* Canad. Med. Assoc. J. **85,** 1136
5. Editorial (1970). *Paracervical block in labour*, Brit. J. Anaes. **42,** 657
6. Doughty A (1969). *Selective Epidural Analgesia and the Forceps Rate*, Brit. J. Anaesth. **41,** 1058.
7. Frumin M J, Schwartz H, Burns J J, Brodie B B and Papper E M (1953). *The Appearance of Procaine in the Spinal Fluid during Peridural Block in Man.* J. Pharmacol. **109,** 102

Acknowledgements
Fig. 1 reproduced by permission from Practical Management of Pain in Labour (1953) by W. D. Wylie. Lloyd-Luke, London.
Fig. 3 reproduced by permission from A Practice of Anaesthesia (3rd edit. 1972) by W. D. Wylie and H. C. Churchill-Davidson. Lloyd-Luke, London.

DISCUSSION

Dr Crawford (Birmingham): I would like to make a couple of comments with reference to the neuroanatomy. I think, from what I gather from Bonica's book[1] and elsewhere, that we can now say fairly confidently that the fibres which convey sensory impulses from the uterus are somatic, although they accompany the sympathetic nerves. We can discount any contribution from the parasympathetic system to uterine sensation. Pain

13

during the second stage of labour is a combination of pain from the contracting uterus and pain of pelvic floor distension, this latter being transmitted via somatic sensory fibres having their central connection at the level of S2, 3, 4 segments.

The Chairman: Are you saying that the pelvic splanchnic nerves probably have no role in the transmission of painful impulses from the uterus?

Dr Crawford (Birmingham): Yes, the 2nd, 3rd and 4th sacral segments are concerned only with the pain of pelvic floor distension.

Dr Colback (Newcastle): I was interested in Dr Doughty's comments. For some time now I have found that volumes of local anaesthetic as low as 3 ml injected at the T12-L1 interspace have abolished labour pain whether felt in the lower abdomen or in the back. In one case the block extended to the sacral roots and the head was lying on the perineum for a considerable time without the patient or her attendants realizing it. I have also had experience of two cases when attempts to achieve a sacral spread of analgesia for forceps delivery was unsuccessful, and in one a subsequent caudal injection to remedy this was also ineffective. I feel therefore that the question of how labour pain is mediated is still very much a matter for debate.

Dr Bryson (Liverpool): In Liverpool we employ the same type of technique as Dr Colback in Newcastle using minimal amounts of local anaesthetic agents to minimise the major complications of epidurals consistent with providing adequate analgesia. Occasionally we have had some difficulty in providing perineal analgesia, but this has been usually due to malposition of the epidural catheter, or to insufficient time being allowed for the local anaesthetic to reach the sacral roots by gravity. Five to ten minutes in the sitting position are required for this. If we do not achieve adequate perineal analgesia, we would rather fault our technique than question the anatomical distribution of the sacral nerves.

Dr Tunstall (Aberdeen): The parasympathetic afferents S2, 3 and 4 in animals play a role in Ferguson's reflex whereby the pituitary is stimulated. This has not been shown to be the case in human beings, but it is likely that they take part in the reflex whereby stimulation of the pelvic parasympathetic causes increased uterine activity.

Dr Burn (Southampton): Dr Doughty questioned the mechanism by which the block in the lumbar region spreads to the sacral region. I do not think that this is due to transdural diffusion to the cerebrospinal fluid affecting the cauda equina, but it is almost certainly a gravity effect, the local anaesthetic solution descending from the lumbar epidural space to the sacral epidural space. We have done a fairly large number of epidurograms recently and have found that these solutions spread easily both up and down the epidural space according to the posture of the patient.

I would like Dr Doughty to 'lay a ghost' about the motor innervation of the uterus. It has been believed for a long time that if the epidural block spreads higher than T10 there is a risk of affecting the course of labour. Many of us are certain that our blocks have spread higher than this and there has been no adverse influence on uterine action. Once labour is

14

established the uterine contractions are not under the influence of the sympathetic supply from T5-10 but entirely under hormonal control.

Dr Doughty (in reply): It is now generally recognised that utero-motor activity is almost totally under hormonal control, but it has been shown that if a block spreading higher than T10 results in a substantial fall of blood pressure, the uterine contractions diminish. If the blood pressure is maintained, the uterine contractions remain as they were before the epidural injection[2].

Dr Crawford (Birmingham): I think Dr Doughty is quite right. I do not believe that uterine activity is reduced for any more than 20 minutes following the injection of fluid into the epidural space which I think is a fairly well recognised response.[2] You cannot reduce uterine activity by introducing a block even as high as T2 once labour has become established. The effect of a high block on uterine activity is only in relation to the premonitory stage of labour. Once labour has become established it is primarily under hormonal control and the other factors have no influence at all. No type of analgesia has an undesirable influence upon the course of labour provided that it does not produce hypotension. On the contrary, if the patient is suffering from severe pain and distress, it is not unusual for the progress of labour to be slowed—presumably as a result partly of the outpouring of catecholamines—and under such circumstances the provision of adequate analgesia will be followed by a return to a normally-progressing labour. *L / T12 block – no adrenal catechols.*

The Chairman: Dr Moir emphasised in the paper that he wrote with Mr Willocks[3] that the severe back pain associated with inco-ordinate action of the uterus was best managed by a sit-up sacral block. Does he still adhere to that view or can it be coped with equally effectively by a small volume block, mid-lumbar, with the patient lying on her side?

Dr Moir (Glasgow): I would be unrepentant on this. I still see patients in whom backache persists with an initial dose of 6 ml given horizontally. A further 2 or 3 ml given in the sitting position will relieve the backache within 5 minutes in this type of labour, the so-called hypertonic inco-ordinate labour and labour in association with occipito-posterior positions. I think that it is often, perhaps not invariably, necessary to block the sacral roots to relieve this backache which is the more severe of the pains which the patient may experience.

REFERENCES

1. Bonica J J (1967). *Principles and Practice of Obstetric Analgesia and Anaesthesia*, Vol. **1**, p.110 Blackwell Scientific Publications, Oxford

2. Vasicka A and Kretchmer N (1961). *Effect of Conduction and Inhalational Anesthesia on Uterine Contractions.* Amer. J. Obstet. Gynec. **82**, 600

3. Moir D D and Willocks J (1967). *Management of Inco-ordinate Uterine Action under Continuous Epidural Analgesia.* Brit. med. J. **3**, 396

The Effect of Continuous Lumbar Epidural Block on Maternal and Foetal Acid-Base Balance During Labour and at Delivery (A Preliminary Report)

Mr J F Pearson (Birmingham)

With the increasing use of continuous lumbar epidural analgesia in labour it is of great importance to know the effect of such a regime of pain relief on the welfare of the mother and child. There has been little work published concerning the effect of epidural block upon materno-foetal acid-base relationships. A preliminary report on the initial findings of such an investigation is presented here:

Material and Methods

From detailed records of 120 personally monitored cases, 26 were selected as conforming to the following criteria of the Clinically Acceptable Ideal Case as originally described by Crawford (1965)[1].

The primigravidae were below the age of 25 years.

The multigravidae were below the age of 35 years.

There was no evidence of obstetrical or medical disorder.

The gestational age at the time of labour was between 38 and 41 weeks.

All cases of nuchal cord were excluded from the study.

In addition, all patients who were given hypertonic fructose infusions during labour to treat ketosis were also excluded, as this procedure induces marked metabolic acidosis in both mother and foetus (Pearson & Shuttleworth, 1971)[2].

Each infant was a singleton cephalic presentation, with Apgar Scores of 9 or 10 at 1 minute.

Labour was monitored by means of the cervimetric charts of Friedman (1955)[3] and each labour selected conforms to the values for normal labour which he describes.

The method of study was as follows:

Maternal arterial blood and foetal scalp blood was taken anaerobically as nearly as possible simultaneously, the maternal arterial blood being taken before a contraction and the scalp sample during the course of a contraction to obviate, as far as possible, minute to minute variations, and to improve sample comparability. Acid-base values were obtained using the Astrup micro-electrode technique[4], the results being derived from the Siggaard-Anderson nomogram[5], with corrections for ambient barometric pressure and oxygen saturation (Radiometer O.S.M.I.). Maternal arterial lactate was measured (following immediate deproteinisation in 0.6% perchloric acid) by the lactate dehydrogenase method of the Boehringer Corporation.

The first sample was taken before the onset of labour and the second sample was taken to coincide as closely as possible with the beginning of the active phase of labour, as indicated on the cervimetric chart; the differences between the two samples being an index of the changes taking place during the latent phase of labour. A third sample was taken at full dilatation and a final sample of maternal arterial blood was taken at crowning. Cord blood was taken from the baby before the first gasp.

At the Birmingham Maternity Hospital it is customary to stimulate uterine contractions by the use of Syntocinon infusion if labour is not established within 4 hours of admission and this practice was adhered to in these cases.

Of the 26 patients, 9 patients comprise the Control group, that is those who did not have an epidural block. The Control group were given the usual conventional analgesia of pethidine 100 mg with or without 25 mg promazine as indicated. None of the Control group received inhalational analgesia during labour.

Seventeen of the patients received continuous epidural analgesia and were pain-free throughout labour, the block being instituted from the beginning of labour. No patient who showed evidence of an incomplete block is included in this report.

Figure 1

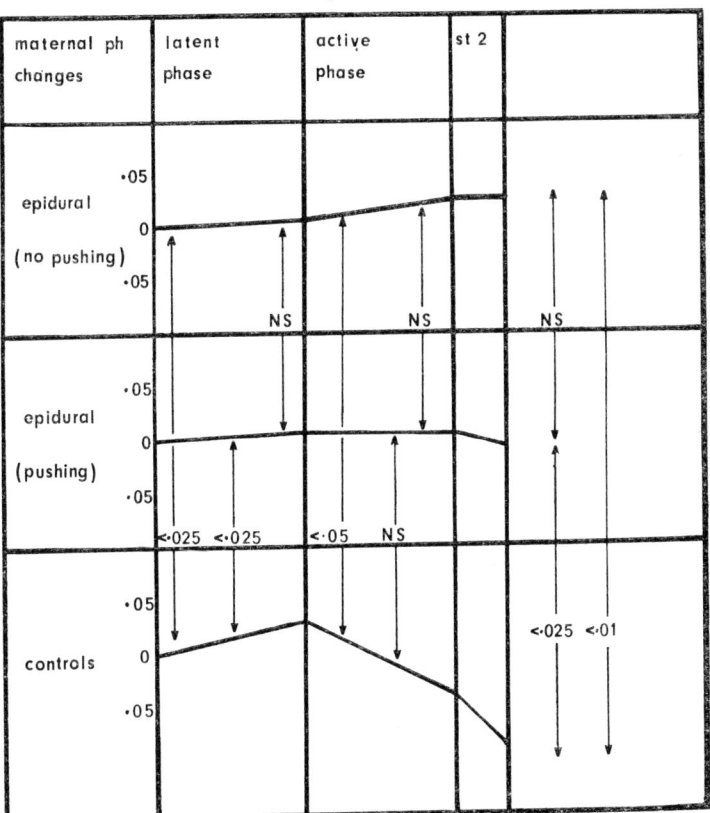

The means of the Maternal Arterial pH changes in labour

These seventeen patients were divided into two groups, the first group (11 patients) consisted of those who retained the urge to push during the second stage despite being rendered pain free. (Epidural-Pushing)

17

The second epidural group (Epidural No-Pushing) consisted of those patients who had no urge to push and were not encouraged to do so. These were delivered by low forceps when the head had descended to the pelvic floor by means of the unaided uterine propulsive forces.

All the patients receiving epidural analgesia were carefully monitored with regard to blood pressure and there were no episodes of hypotension in any of these patients.

Results

Figure 1. This diagram indicates the mean changes of maternal arterial pH during labour and at delivery. Each patient is used as her own control and all values are indicated as deviations from the initial pre-labour value. The significance of the differences between the Control group and the two Epidural groups was calculated by means of Student's t-Test for unpaired differences of means.

Figure 2

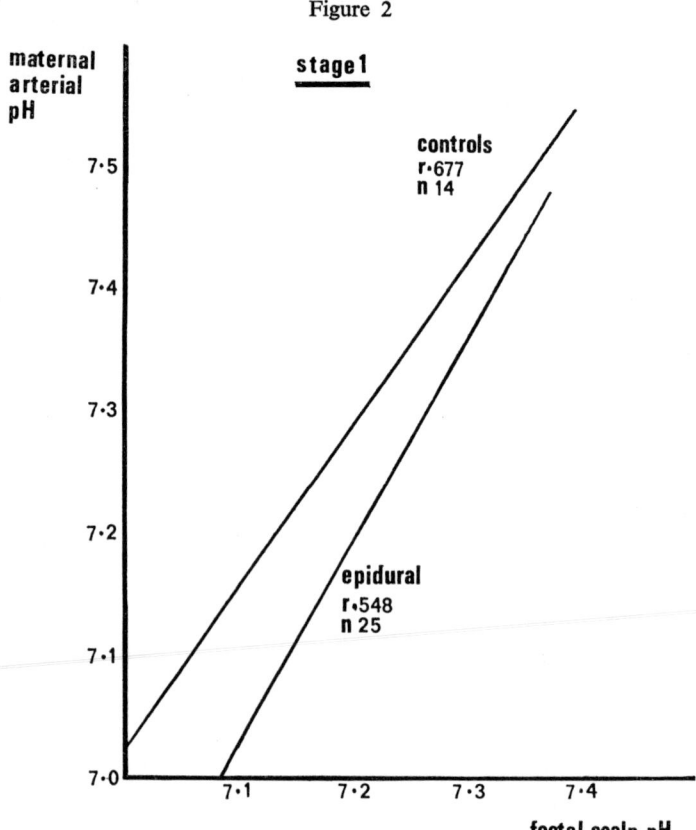

The correlation between Maternal Arterial and Foetal Scalp pH during the First Stage of Labour.

In the Control group there is initially a rise in pH during the latent phase followed during the active phase by a fall in pH with yet a further fall during the second stage of labour.

In both Epidural groups there is little change in maternal arterial pH values during the first stage of labour. During the second stage the fall in maternal arterial pH in the Control group is significantly greater than the pH fall in either Epidural group. The difference between the two Epidural groups with respect to the change in maternal arterial pH during the second stage is not significant.

The degree of correlation between maternal arterial and foetal scalp pH in the first stage of labour is shown by Figure 2. Reasonably good correlation exists in both groups of patients and there is no obvious difference between them.

Figure 3

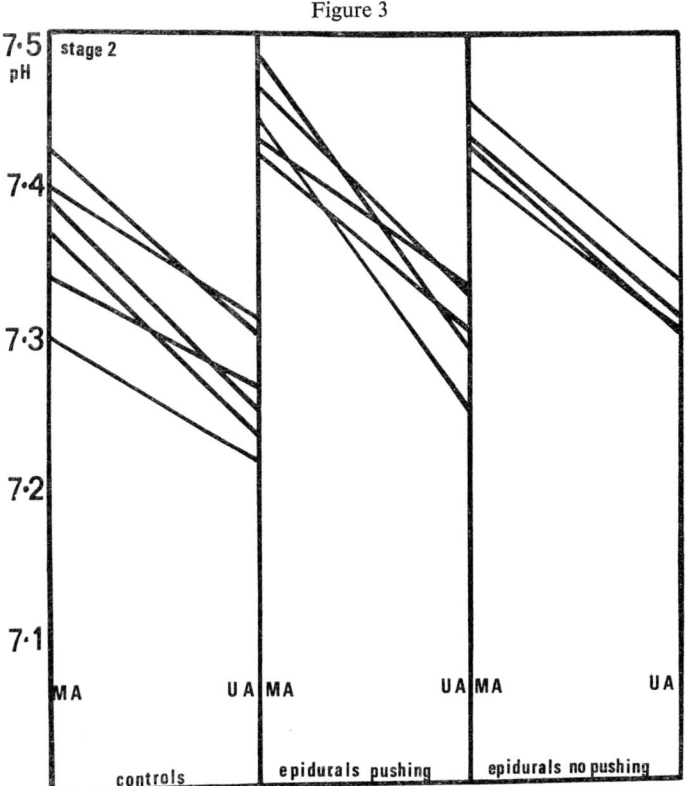

The Maternal Arterial (MA): Umbilical Arterial (UA) relationships of pH at the time of delivery in the three groups of patients.

The next diagram (Figure 3) represents the Maternal Arterial: Umbilical Arterial pH gradient existing at the time of delivery in terms of their absolute values. The umbilical arterial pH in all groups is lower than the maternal arterial pH but the maternal arterial pH is higher in the Epidural groups than in the Control group.

Figure 4

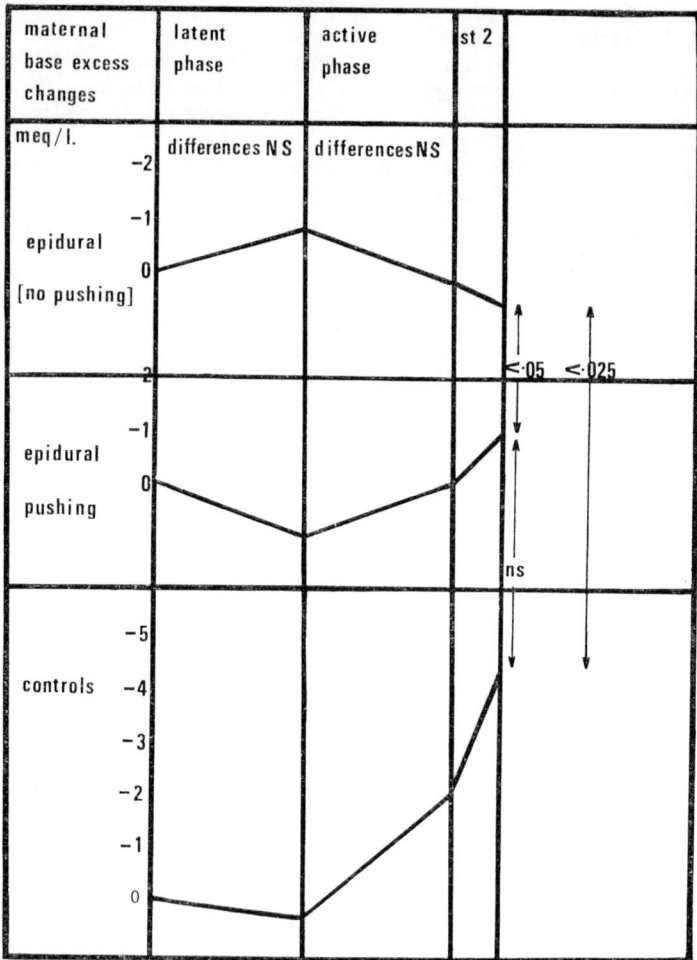

The means of the Maternal Arterial Base Excess changes during labour.

Figure 4. With regard to Maternal arterial base-excess changes during labour, there is no statistically significant difference between the Epidural groups and the Control group during the first stage of labour, although there does appear to be a trend towards an increased metabolic acidosis in the Control group during the Active Phase. During the second stage of labour there is a marked metabolic acidosis in the Control group. In the Epidural group who were pushing during the second stage, there is an increase in metabolic acidosis which is of smaller degree than the Controls but of greater degree than the Epidural group who did not push and who showed no tendency towards metabolic acidosis.

Figure 5

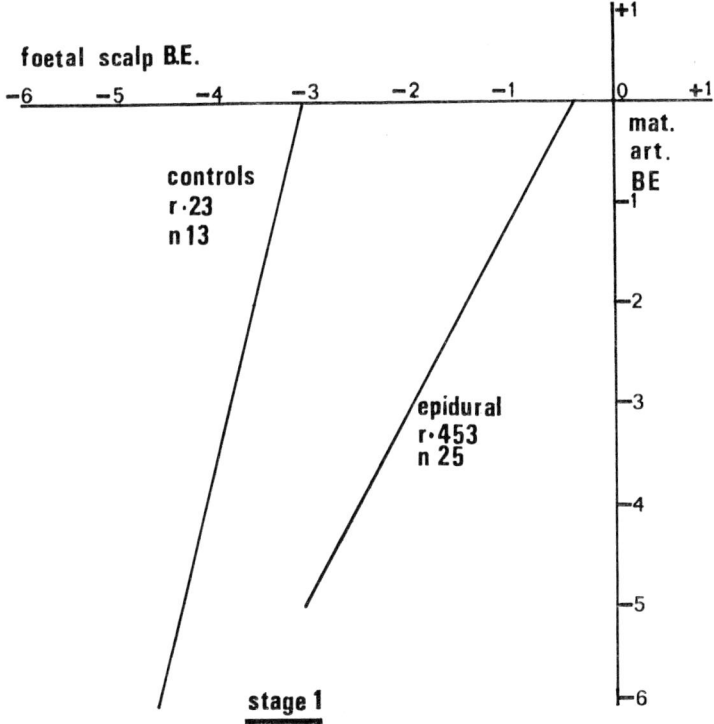

The correlation between Maternal and Arterial and Foetal Scalp Base Excess during the First Stage of Labour.

Figure 5. This diagram illustrates the correlation between maternal arterial and foetal scalp base excess during the first stage of labour. Although good correlation exists in the two Epidural groups, only poor correlation exists in the Control group. This poor correlation is reflective of the findings presented in Figure 6 which depicts the changes in foetal scalp base excess during labour using the same diagrammatic convention as in Figure 4. In the Control group of foetuses there is an increase in base excess during the latent phase which, although it follows the overall pattern of the mother, (see Figure 4) is of much greater extent than one would expect on the basis of simple Maternal-Foetal infusion. I am unable to offer an explanation for this phenomenon. If it were due to an improvement in foetal oxygenation reflecting increased placental perfusion as a result of myometrial activity, one would expect the same phenomenon to occur in the foetuses of the Epidural groups. However, the foetuses of the Epidural groups seem to show the same lack of variation of base excess as do their mothers during the first stage of labour. There is, during the second stage of labour, an increased base deficit in all three groups of foetuses in marked contrast to the maternal situation in the Epidural groups. The

21

Figure 6

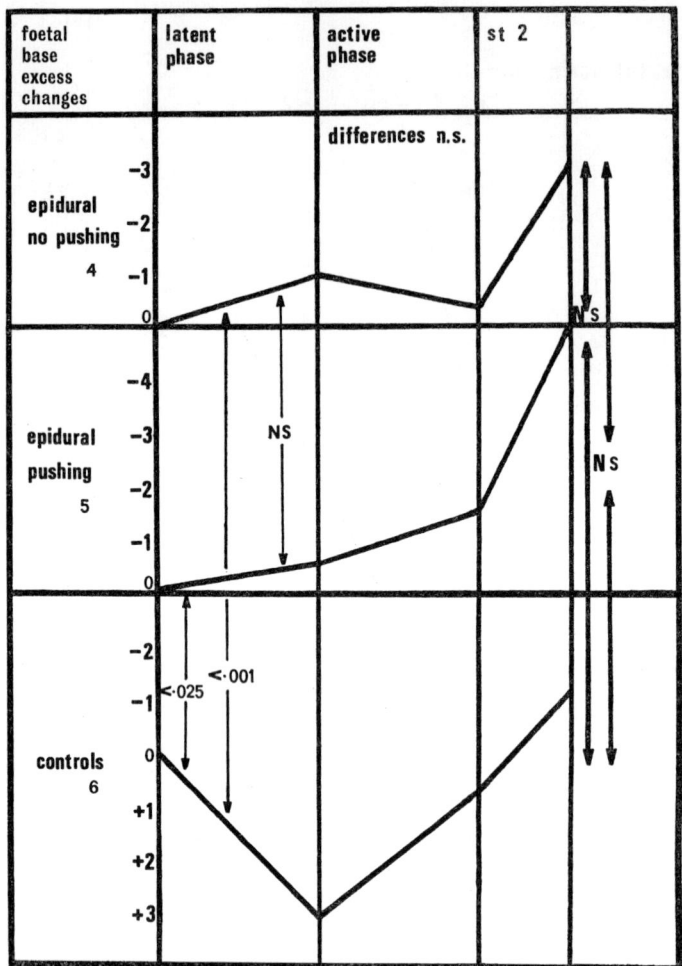

The means of the changes in Foetal Scalp Base Excess during Labour.

most likely explanation for this notable event is that the foetus experiences a degree of metabolic acidosis during the second stage of labour which is, to a large extent, independent of the mother's acid-base state and is likely to be consequent upon and reflective of, a degree of impaired placental perfusion associated with the increased uterine retraction taking place as the body of the uterus empties. In support of this explanation the mean duration of the second stage in the Control group who experienced both pain and a strong urge to push was 23 minutes, the Epidural group who were pushing painlessly spent 59 minutes in the second stage and in the Epidural group who were not pushing the mean duration of the second stage was 64 minutes. It thus appears that the foetus will incrementally

22

accumulate base deficit throughout the second stage of labour, independently of the maternal acid-base situation.

Figure 7

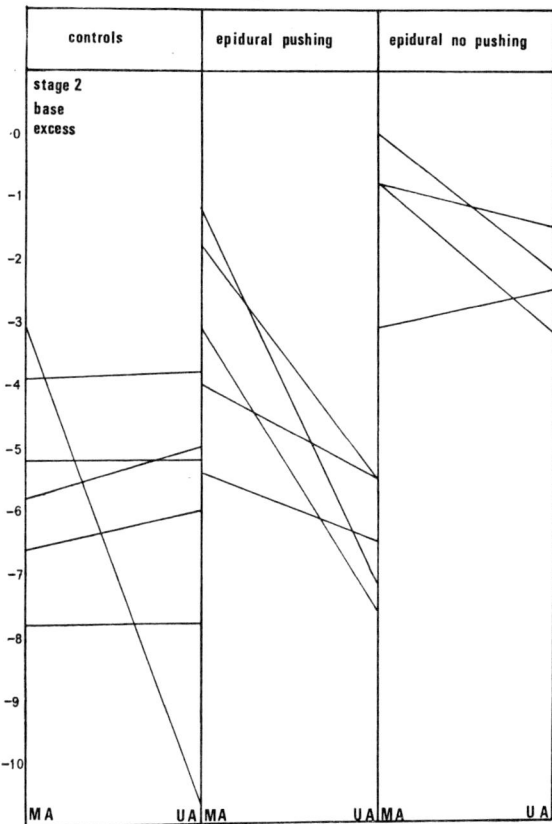

The Maternal Arterial (MA) and Umbilical Arterial (UA) Base Excess relationships at the time of delivery.

Figure 7. This diagram illustrates the relationship between maternal arterial base excess and umbilical arterial base excess at delivery.

In the Control group, with one exception, there is little difference in base excess values which reflects:

(a) the fall in maternal base excess during the second stage.

(b) the smaller degree of fall of foetal base excess in this group which is related to the shorter second stage.

In both Epidural groups there is a considerable difference between maternal arterial and umbilical arterial base excess at delivery reflecting:

(a) The small change in maternal base excess during the second stage—especially in the non-pushing group.

(b) The greater degree of foetal metabolic acidosis occurring in the foetus as a result of the more prolonged second stage.

23

Figure 8

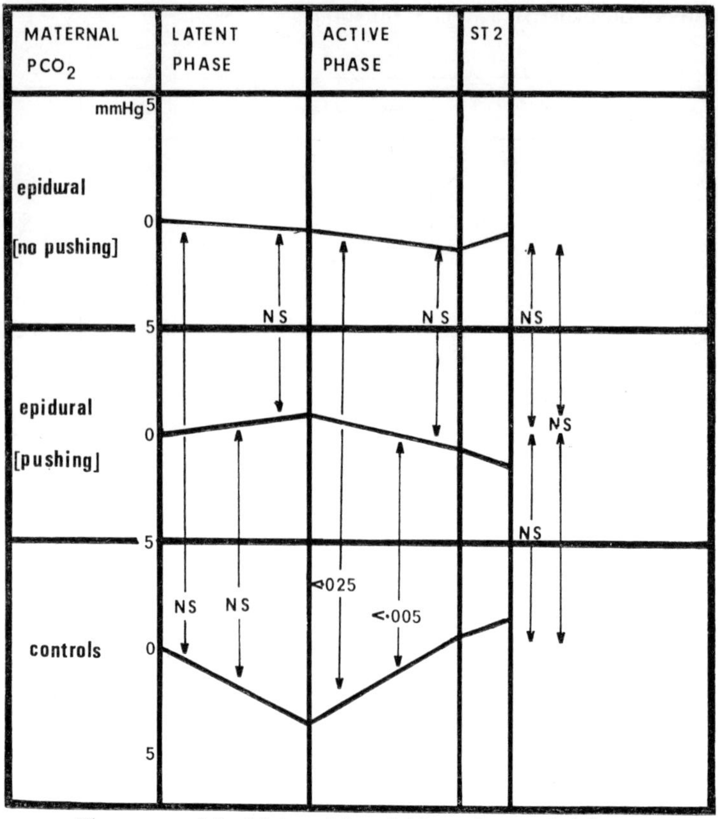

MATERNAL PCO_2	LATENT PHASE	ACTIVE PHASE	ST 2	

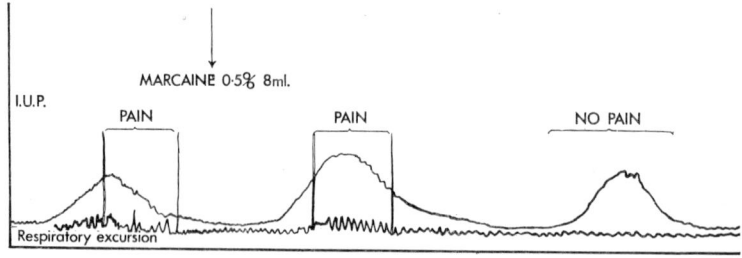

The means of the Maternal Arterial Pco_2 changes in labour.

Figure 8. The maternal Pco_2 changes are indicated in this diagram. In the Control series a respiratory alkalosis develops during the latent phase due to hyperventilation. This appears to be in response to pain, as

Figure 9

MARCAINE 0·5% 8ml.

I.U.P.

PAIN   PAIN   NO PAIN

Respiratory excursion

The effect of relief on Maternal respiratory performance during painful and painless contractions.

women in both Epidural groups show little change in PCO_2 levels. During the second stage there is an increase in PCO_2 which is reflective of:

(a) Increased CO_2 production as a result of increased energy expenditure.

(b) Breath-holding during expulsive efforts during the second stage.

Evidence in support of the contention that the hyperventilation in early labour is due to pain is offered in Figure 9 which shows the maternal respiratory excursion (as measured by a tambour on the sternum) related to intra-uterine pressure as recorded by an intra-uterine pressure transducer. The patient herself was able to mark the recording paper by pressing a switch at the onset of pain and again when the pain disappeared. The recording shows that pain relief is associated with a return to normal respiratory excursion. It is notable that the duration of the hyperventilation closely approximates to the period of time during which pain was experienced. Figure 10 shows the close correlation between maternal arterial and foetal scalp PCO_2 in both groups of patients.

Figure 10

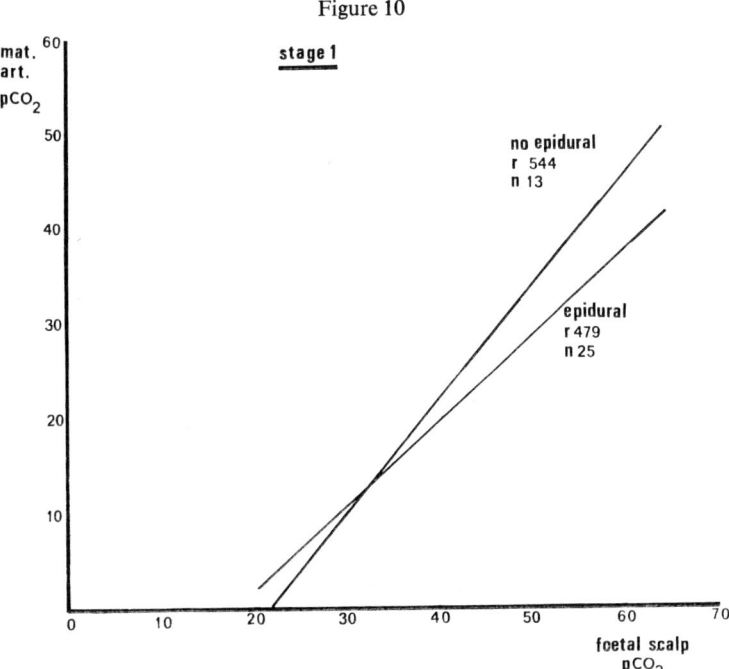

The correlation between Maternal Arterial PCO_2 and Foetal Scalp PCO_2

With regard to maternal lactate accumulation in the mother, it is generally accepted that this is likely to be due to the results of anaerobic glycogen metabolism occurring during muscular activity. The source of lactate in labour may therefore be skeletal or uterine muscle. If the main source of lactate accumulation in labour was uterine muscle a similar incremental increase in the concentration of lactate should occur equally

25

Figure 11

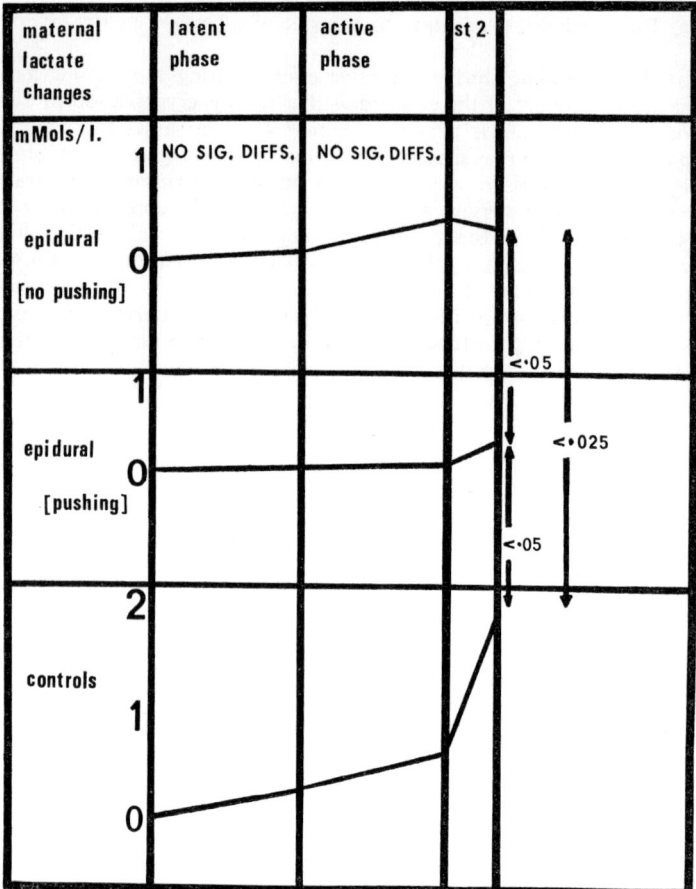

The Means of the Maternal Arterial Lactate changes in labour.

in all three groups of patients especially during the active phase. Although not statistically significant there is a larger mean increase in the concentration of lactate in the women of the Control group than those of the Epidural groups (Figure 11).

The striking increase in lactate concentration in women of the Control group during the second stage of labour is significantly greater than in either Epidural group; whilst those patients with an epidural block who were pushing produced more lactate than those who did not push.

One can, therefore, reasonably conclude that women without epidural analgesia are able to push more strongly than those with such analgesia— a proposition which is supported by the findings of a much shorter second stage in the Control group.

A study of the effect of lumbar epidural analgesia on the acid base balance of normal parturient women has been presented.

In normal labour there is maternal respiratory alkalosis during the latent phase of the first stage which is abolished during the active phase and the second stage of labour.

Women given epidural analgesia throughout labour showed little deviation in P_{CO_2} from the pre-labour values. The maternal P_{CO_2} levels were closely correlated with those of the foetus at all stages of labour.

Plethysmographic evidence supports the contention that hyperventilation plays a part in the physiological response to pain as this response is abolished by the institution of epidural blockade.

In the control series there was a slight tendency towards metabolic alkalosis during the latent phase of labour followed by progressive maternal metabolic acidosis which reached its maximum towards the end of the second stage.

In contrast, the epidural groups showed no deviation from the pre-labour values throughout the first stage of labour. During the second stage the group who were pushing became more acidotic due to the products of skeletal muscular activity in the same manner as did the controls. This observation supports the contention that the metabolic acidosis in normal labour may depend more upon the metabolites of skeletal muscle than of uterine muscle. This is almost certainly so in the second stage of labour when one contrasts the metabolic acidosis produced in the group who were pushing, with the more 'steady state' obtained in the group who were not pushing.

The overall pattern of change in the foetus depends in general on maternal-foetal perfusion. However, during the second stage of labour it was evident that the infants of all three groups of patients developed a metabolic acidosis, the degree of severity depending on the duration of the second stage rather than the degree of maternal acidosis. This effect was most marked in the epidural group electively delivered by forceps who had the longest second stages and also the least change of maternal acid base state during this period of time. This emphasises the importance of ascertaining full cervical dilatation by frequent examination of the patient towards the end of the first stage, and of limiting the length of the second stage to some degree. However, on the basis of available data it is not possible to define an optimum period of time, especially in those cases in which there is pre-existing obstetric abnormality. This aspect is, however, at present being investigated by the writer.

The maternal concentration of lactate follows the overall pattern shown by base excess, the concentration of lactate being especially increased during the second stage of labour. Lactate accumulation in the mother is consequent upon muscular activity. The mean durations of the second stages were longest in the epidural no-pushing group, the shortest in the control group. It can be seen that in the control group there was the largest increase in lactate and that the smallest increase in lactate was in the epidural no-pushing group. One is able to deduce that women without epidural analgesia are able to push harder and more effectively than those

27

with an epidural block, with the consequent benefit of a shorter second stage and hence a diminished level of foetal acidosis.

However, one must point out that although the increased length of the second stage may cause increased metabolic acidosis in the foetus, it has also shown that the 'epidural' foetuses *commence* the second stage in a less acidotic state than the control foetuses but that at delivery they all appear to be similar in acid base status.

In order to obtain optimum results, especially in 'at risk' cases, one would suggest that epidural analgesia can be recommended as being beneficial to the foetus as long as the duration of second stage is limited with respect to time. This would seem to be the form of management of labour which has the least deleterious effect upon the infant.

REFERENCES

1. Crawford J S (1955). *Maternal and Cord Blood at Delivery. Parameters of Respiratory Exchange.* Biol. Neonat. **8**, 131

2. Pearson J F and Shuttleworth R (1971). *The Metabolic Effects of a Hypertonic Fructose Infusion on the Mother and Fetus during Labor.* Amer. J. Obstet. Gyec. **iii**, 259

3. Friedman E A (1955). *Primigravid Labor - a graphico-statistical analysis.* Obstet. Gynec. **6**, 567

4. Astrup P, Jørgensen K, Siggaard-Anderson O and Engel K (1960). *The Acid-base Metabolism: A New Approach.* Lancet **1**, 1035

5. Siggaard-Anderson O and Engel K (1960). *A Micro-method for Determination of pH, Carbon-dioxide Tension, Base Excess and Standard Bicarbonate in Capillary Blood.* Scand. J. Clin. Lab. Invest. **12**, 172

Acknowledgements

I wish to thank the Endowment Fund of the United Birmingham Hospitals for financial assistance, the Department of Anaesthetics of the Birmingham Maternity Hospital for the use of technical equipment. I wish to express my thanks to the Consultant staff of the Birmingham Maternity Hospital whose patients were investigated, to Dr Selwyn Crawford for his advice and criticism, to Mrs M Smith for the preparation of the typescript, to Mr D Williams for the preparation of the illustrations, to Mrs I Brown for statistical assistance and in particular to Miss Aviet and the nursing staff of the Main Delivery Suite, without whose help and co-operation this study could not have been undertaken.

DISCUSSION

Dr Colback (Newcastle): You showed very clearly that, with the relief of pain, uterine contractions no longer caused the mother to hyperventilate. Nevertheless I have noticed on several occasions that the tired patient, while getting complete relief from an epidural, even falling asleep, may yet still obviously hyperventilate during contractions. I am thinking of one particular patient with severe cardiac disease who not only had a completely effective epidural but was under light to medium trance hypnosis. Before induction of labour her haemoglobin was 18·5 grams per cent and, breathing air, her P_{AO_2} was 59 mm.Hg. During labour, breathing oxygen at 6 l/min by M.C. mask, her P_{AO_2} fell to 46 mm.Hg. I can only infer that the oxygen requirement of the contracting uterus produced a respiratory drive despite the relief of pain. Would you like to comment?

Mr Pearson (in reply): It is difficult to comment on the individual case. This is especially difficult when one attempts to extrapolate findings on my Clinically Acceptable Ideal series to a patient with cardiac disease of some severity as judged from the haemoglobin and oxygen saturation levels.

Normally an increased PCO_2 rather than oxygen lack is the major stimulus to respiration in the adult human being. There is no doubt that the work done by the contracting uterus will transiently increase CO_2 production, and if the PCO_2 rose to a high enough level a reflex increase in ventilation would result. My main contention is that, although uterine activity remains constant, the involuntary respiratory performance is altered by pain, but when pain is relieved, despite similar uterine activity, the respiratory pattern remains essentially unchanged.

Dr Bryson (Liverpool): Do your findings suggest that we should be more critical of smaller falls in scalp blood pH as indicating foetal distress in women who have epidurals than in those who do not?

Mr Pearson (in reply): I would agree that any fall of pH which is *independent* of the maternal arterial pH would indicate foetal acidosis, and as the range of maternal arterial pH in those cases who have epidurals is small, one is able to detect foetal anoxia at an earlier stage. However, one seldom sees a depressed infant at birth if the scalp pH is above 7·25 whether or not the mother has had epidural analgesia.

Professor Simpson (London Hospital): I should like to congratulate Mr Pearson on a beautiful piece of work and ask him if there is any correlation between the foetal heart rate and the progressive metabolic acidosis which he has seen in the foetuses of patients subjected to epidural.

Mr Pearson (in reply): Although we have done some studies with combined foetal scalp samples and foetal ECG recordings, we have been unable to demonstrate any consistent change in rate or rhythm of the foetal heart with regard to the progressive foetal acidosis which occurs in normal labour. In cases where infants are severely depressed, the usual ECG signs (which have been well studied elsewhere) are seen, but the degree of acidosis in such cases is far more severe than anything I have presented today.

Dr Hargrove (Westminster Hospital): I also would congratulate Mr Pearson on the research but I am a little disturbed at successive arterial punctures in otherwise normal individuals and I would like to ask him what he feels concerning the ethical position about doing this sort of research on patients where the research itself does not contribute at all to their treatment.

Mr Pearson (in reply): All patients in the above series freely gave permission, having clearly understood what was involved. There is a considerable body of opinion supporting the contention that arterial puncture is a very safe procedure.

Mr Noble (Westminster Hospital): I would like to add my congratulations to Mr Pearson on this interesting study. At the Westminster Hospital, our findings regarding the length of the second stage of labour accord with his. His finding of a relative and increasing foetal metabolic acidosis during this time should make us cautious when the foetus is at special risk—for example the dysmature foetus.

We also have studied foetal and neonatal welfare in relation to epidural analgesia; our results are of interest and complementary to his findings. Our patients were selected in a manner similar to his and we studied foetal heart tracings, foetal pH whenever there were clinical signs of foetal distress and umbilical artery pH at birth; we also noted the 5-minute Apgar score. We compared 100 patients with epidural analgesia with 102 women who had either routine narcotic analgesia or no analgesia at all. Instrumental delivery was performed for foetal distress or for failure to progress. In our study the babies in the epidural group fared better; they had higher pH recordings and higher Apgar scores, there was no difference in the incidence of foetal distress.

We believe that epidural analgesia offers advantages for the foetus when associated with good standards of clinical practice. Avoidance of an over-long second stage and indeed the early diagnosis of this stage are important points. Mr Pearson has made a notable contribution.

The Influence of Adrenaline on Maternal and Neonatal Blood Levels of Local Analgesic Drugs

DR FELICITY REYNOLDS (St Thomas's Hospital, London)

The practice of continuous epidural analgesia in labour may, if prolonged, lead to rather large doses of local analgesic drug's being given, and consequently can involve the risk of systemic toxicity from the drug. In order to assess the possible accumulation of drugs in the systemic circulation and to predict the dangers of toxicity, it is necessary to measure blood concentrations of local analgesics after successive epidural doses. Any blood level will be the resultant of absorption into and elimination from the circulation and is not a function only of dosage. Other factors are the vascularity of the site of injection and the extent to which this may have been altered by the local analgesic drug itself (some have vasoconstrictor and others vasodilator properties) or by the addition of adrenaline, which is known to limit the absorption of local analgesic drugs. The third factor which may alter the absorption of the drug is its distribution at the site of the injection between the aqueous phase and the tissues. The more lipid soluble drugs are more taken up in tissues, whereas with the less lipid soluble ones a higher proportion remains in the aqueous phase for absorption into the circulation.

Figure 1

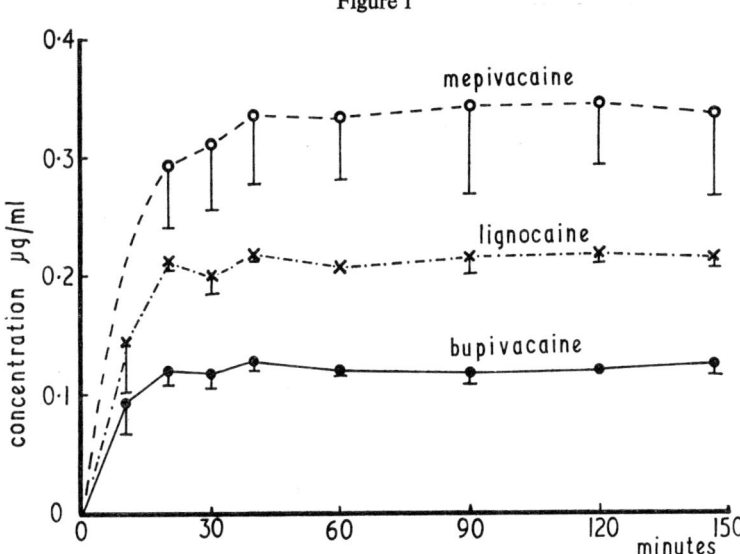

Mean blood concentrations of local analgesic drugs in surgical patients, each of whom was given a single epidural injection containing equal doses of all three with adrenaline. Vertical lines represent standard errors. (n = 3)

Figure 1 shows that blood concentration is not purely a function of dosage. In this figure a group of patients was given a mixture of 0.25% bupivacaine (Marcain), 0.25% lignocaine and 0.25% mepivacaine (Carbo-

31

caine), yet it is quite clear that bupivacaine gave rise to much the lowest blood concentrations and mepivacaine the highest. When the same mixture was given in 10 ml doses two-hourly to maintain analgesia in labour, the same differences in blood concentration were seen, but as labour progressed the differences were magnified, and by the end of labour bupivacaine had accumulated little and mepivacaine quite markedly.

These three drugs are, of course, of different potencies, and they have been given in the mixture at a dosage rate akin to that of bupivacaine alone. It is perhaps of greater clinical relevance to compare their cumulative tendencies when each is given at a dosage and frequency sufficient to maintain analgesia by itself. Reynolds and Taylor[1] compared lignocaine and bupivacaine given individually, each with adrenaline, to produce continuous epidural analgesia in labour.

Figure 2

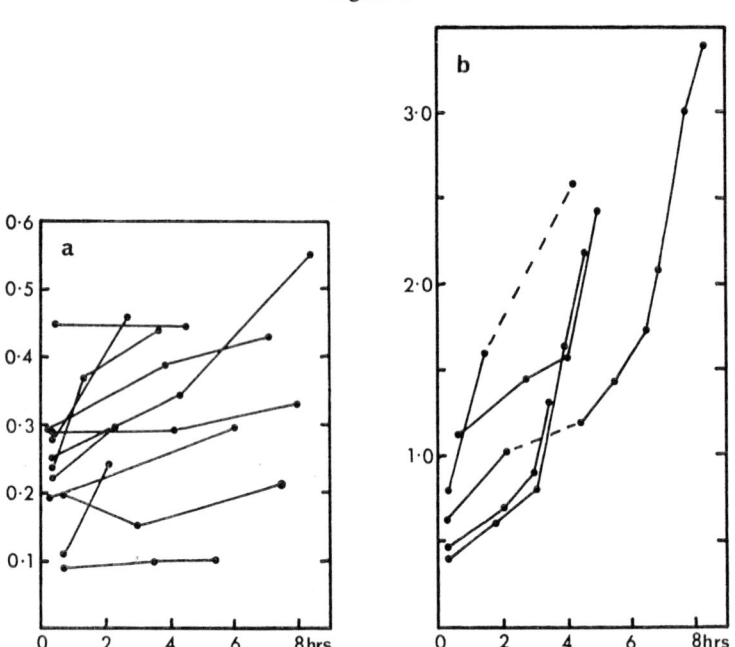

Peak blood concentrations in μg/ml after successive epidural doses of (a) bupivacaine in 11 cases, and (b) lignocaine in 5 cases. Dotted lines indicate omission of samples after a dose.

Figure 2 shows the peak blood concentrations measured after successive epidural doses, in individuals in the two groups. In the case of bupivacaine, peak levels after the final doses were usually only fractionally higher than after the initial doses, whereas with lignocaine, in all cases final concentrations were several times the initial concentrations. Of course lignocaine had to be given much more frequently than bupivacaine. Adrenaline is known to retard the absorption of lignocaine, to reduce its toxicity and to prolong its action, yet its inclusion is unable to prevent the accumulation of lignocaine in the blood.

However, is adrenaline necessary with bupivacaine? Adrenaline is a relatively short acting drug and it is known to increase the potential toxicity of an accidental intravenous injection.[2] Therefore if it is to be included, the indications for its use should be carefully considered. Bupivacaine is a highly lipid soluble drug, it has mild vasoconstrictor properties of its own, it is taken up in the tissues locally to a marked extent, and it is longer acting than adrenaline itself. Although it has been shown that adrenaline marginally increases the duration of action of bupivacaine[3] when used in relatively large doses for anaesthesia in elective surgery, this is probably clinically unimportant. It is therefore of interest to find out if it has any significant effect on small repeated doses used in labour.

Figure 3

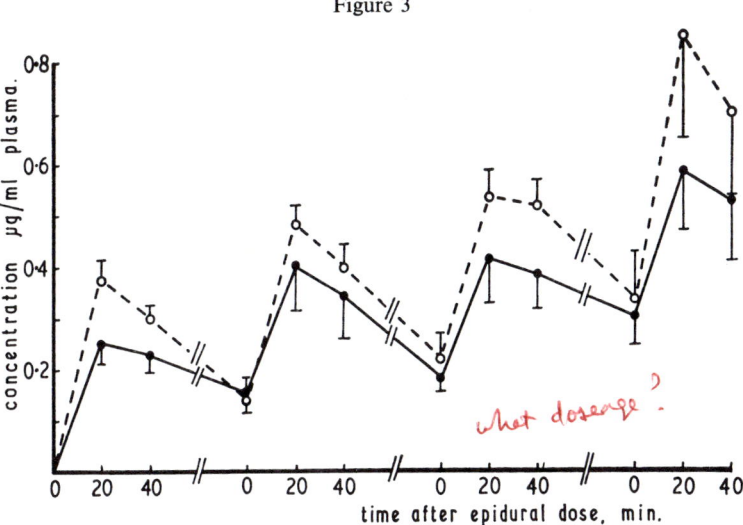

Mean plasma concentrations of bupivacaine after successive epidural doses of bupivacaine alone (o – – – o) and with adrenaline (●————●). Vertical lines represent standard errors.

Two groups of patients were given bupivacaine alone (9 patients) or bupivacaine with adrenaline (9 patients) using a double blind technique.[4] It was found that adrenaline did not increase the duration of action of bupivacaine in this particular series. Therefore it was possible to compare the blood concentrations in the two groups, both before and 20 and 40 minutes after each successive dose of bupivacaine (Figure 3). All patients received two doses of bupivacaine and thereafter fewer patients required further doses. For those who did so, many doses were larger in order to maintain analgesia in late labour. Although adrenaline slightly reduces the plasma concentration 20 and 40 minutes after each dose, when the next dose is due there is, in fact, never a difference worth mentioning between the plasma concentrations in the two groups. Only towards the end of labour, when larger doses are necessary, does adrenaline make a marked difference. The series would need to be larger to show statistical significance. However, it is quite clear that bupivacaine is a drug which is not markedly cumulative in labour whether or not adrenaline is included. I think that one can safely give repeated 30 mg doses to maintain analgesia in labour for as long as necessary. When larger doses are required for the second stage adrenaline should probably be included, to reduce the danger of bupivacaine toxicity.

Placental transfer of local analgesic drugs

The placenta is a barrier to charged particles: ions in normal conditions will not cross the placenta, but lipid soluble substances up to a molecular weight of 600–1,000 can cross and are likely to do so at a rate proportional to the gradient and lipid solubility of the free unionised form of the molecule. Therefore one might expect that the baby's local anaesthetic level will bear a fairly constant relationship to the mother's, given time

Figure 4

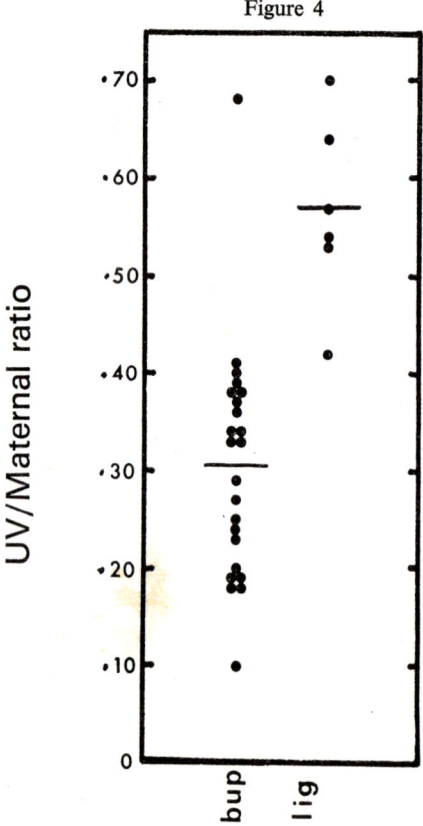

Neonatal (UV) : Maternal blood concentration ratios of bupivacaine (bup) and lignocaine (lig) at delivery, after epidural injection.

34

for equilibration between the two circulations. In order to study this relationship, one can look at the ratio between the umbilical venous (UV) and the maternal venous blood concentrations.

Figure 4 shows the UV: maternal ratios in two groups of patients, one given lignocaine and the other bupivacaine, both with adrenaline. Bupivacaine has a mean UV: maternal ratio of about 0·3, lignocaine 0·5–0·6[5][6] and mepivacaine 0·7[7][8]. Though bupivacaine is the most lipid soluble drug of this group, it does not appear to cross the placenta as readily as the other two drugs. Bupivacaine is highly protein-bound; the concentration of *free* drug in the plasma is thereby lowered. Protein binding thus retards and impedes its placental transfer. Not only therefore are maternal levels of bupivacaine low, but the UV: maternal ratio is also low, when compared to the other drugs. The result of this is that neonatal levels of bupivacaine at delivery are on an average about one-tenth those of lignocaine and one thirtieth those of mepivacaine: a marked difference. This bears out what is found in practice: both lignocaine and mepivacaine have been thought to produce neonatal depression occasionally,[6][7] whereas I do not think that there is good evidence that bupivacaine has ever produced neonatal depression after a correctly administered epidural block.

Table 1

Maternal and UV plasma concentrations at delivery following bupivacaine with and without adrenaline

	Plasma concentration at delivery Mean ± SE. µg/ml		UV: maternal ratio
	maternal	UV	(Mean)
Bupivacaine alone	0·67 ± 0·12	0·16 ± 0·04	0·23
Bupivacaine with adrenaline	0·49 ± 0·08	0·18 ± 0·03	0·40

Adrenaline should only influence neonatal concentrations in so far as it influences maternal concentrations, and one would not expect it to alter placental perfusion or the UV: maternal ratio. However, Table 1 shows maternal and UV plasma concentrations at delivery in two groups of patients, one given bupivacaine alone, and the other bupivacaine with adrenaline. There is no significant difference between the two groups in respect of either maternal or UV concentrations, yet it is clear that the UV: maternal ratio is substantially higher after bupivacaine with adrenaline. This cannot be explained in terms of dose-delivery intervals since these were the same in the two groups.[4] This phenomenon, also experienced with lignocaine,[9][10] is being further investigated. It is clear however that the inclusion of adrenaline with epidural bupivacaine offers no protection to the baby, in whom, anyway, plasma concentrations are habitually low.

Summary

In continuous epidural analgesia, large doses of a local analgesic drug may lead to systemic toxicity in mother or baby. In order to estimate the cumulative tendency of a drug, and therefore its potential systemic toxicity, blood concentrations have been measured after successive epidural injections.

Plasma concentrations of an epidurally administered drug are a resultant of absorption into and elimination from the circulation, and therefore not wholly dependent on dosage. Thus, when bupivacaine, lignocaine and mepivacaine are given in equal doses, blood levels of bupivacaine are lower than those of lignocaine and much lower than those of mepivacaine.

Adrenaline prolongs the action and delays the absorption of many local analgesic drugs, yet it does increase the toxicity of an accidental intravenous injection. Thus indications for its use should be carefully assessed.

Adrenaline significantly reduces lignocaine absorption and prolongs its action, yet it is unable to prevent marked accumulation of lignocaine used for prolonged epidural analgesia. Bupivacaine on the other hand is more lipid soluble and less cumulative, with vaso-constrictor properties of its own and a longer duration of action; adrenaline has a negligible effect on both duration and toxicity of bupivacaine in small repeated doses.

Placental transfer of a local analgesic drug depends on the gradient and lipid solubility of the free unionised portion. Bupivacaine, which is highly protein bound, has an umbilical cord/maternal blood concentration ratio at delivery of about 0·3, compared to lignocaine 0·5–0·6 and mepivacaine 0·7. Concentrations of bupivacaine at birth are about a tenth those of lignocaine and a thirtieth those of mepivacaine, and do not appear to be associated with neonatal depression. The use of adrenaline has less effect on neonatal than on maternal concentrations of bupivacaine and lignocaine. It is hard to see how adrenaline, in small epidural doses, can influence placental transfer of a local analgesic drug.

REFERENCES

1. Reynolds F and Taylor G (1970). *Maternal and neonatal concentrations of bupivacaine: a comparison with lignocaine during continuous extradural analgesia.* Anaesthesia, **25**, 14

2. Henn F and Brattsand R (1966). *Some pharmacological and toxicological properties of a new long-acting local analgesic LAC-43 (Marcaine), in comparison with mepivacaine and tetracaine.* Acta anaesth. Scandinav. Supplement, **21**, 9

3. Waters H R, Rosen N and Perkins D H (1970). *Extradural blockade with bupivacaine. A double blind trial of bupivacaine with adrenaline 1/200,000 and bupivacaine plain.* Anaesthesia, **25**, 184

4. Reynolds F and Taylor G (1971). *Plasma concentrations of bupivacaine during continuous epidural analgesia in labour: the effect of adrenaline.* Brit. J. Anaesth. **43**, 436

5. Shnider S M and Way E L (1968). *Plasma levels of lidocaine (Xylocaine[R]) in mother and newborn following obstetrical conduction anesthesia.* Anesthesiology, **29**, 951

6. Thomas J, Climie C R and Mather L E (1968). *Placental transfer of lignocaine following lumbar epidural administration.* Brit. J. Anaesth. **40**, 965

7. Morishima H O, Daniel S S, Finster M, Poppers P J and James L S (1966). *Transmission of mepivacaine across the human placenta.* Anesthesiology, **27**, 147

8. Moore D C, Bridenbaugh L D, Bagdi P A and Bridenbaugh P O (1968). *Accumulation of mepivacaine hydrochloride during caudal block.* Anesthesiology, **29**, 585

9. Epstein B S, Banerjee S G and Coakley C S (1968). *Passage of lidocaine and prilocaine across the placenta.* Curr. Res. Anesth. **47**, 223

10. Thomas J, Climie C R, Long G and Nighjoy L E (1969). *The influence of adrenaline on the maternal plasma levels and placental transfer of lignocaine following lumbar epidural administration.* Brit. J. Anaesth. **41**, 1029

Acknowledgements

Figures 2 and 4 are published by permission of the Editor of Anaesthesia: Figure 3 by permission of the Editor of the British Journal of Anaesthesia.

DISCUSSION

The Chairman: Thank you very much Dr Reynolds. Your contribution is very relevant as it is only recently that we have been able to obtain bupivacaine without adrenaline and despite agitation over the past three or four years we have had to accept it pre-mixed with adrenaline. Not only would I like to call for comments on your paper in particular, but also comments on the use of bupivacaine with and without adrenaline, and why we have been unable to obtain the plain solution for so long.

Dr Wilson (Leeds): There was one inconsistency in Figure 3 where you showed rising maternal blood concentrations of bupivacaine whether adrenaline was present or not and these concentrations seemed to rise from zero to 0·8 μg per ml. in the absence of adrenaline. This did not seem to be in line with the rest of your paper. In the paper that you wrote with Gordon Taylor[1] I did not notice rises of this magnitude in the maternal blood concentration.

Dr Reynolds (in reply): Referring to Figure 3, you say that you saw a rise from zero to 0·8 μg per ml. One must always start at zero, but the relative rise of the *peaks* after the first and final doses in individual subjects is not very great. Now we found that to maintain analgesia for the second stage you needed a bigger dose, therefore you would expect a higher peak, and there was a progressive rise in blood concentration due to the fact that some of those patients who contributed to the mean levels were having their final doses.

Dr Wilson: You have ultimately arrived at a peak dose of 0·8 μg per ml which strikes me as rather a high dose verging on the near toxic level.

Dr Reynolds (in reply): No, this was a plasma level. The plasma levels of bupivacaine are almost twice whole blood levels because bupivacaine is highly bound to plasma proteins and therefore very little enters the cells. In my experience the toxic plasma level of bupivacaine is something approaching 2 μg per ml and a plasma level of 0·8 μg per ml after bupivacaine without adrenaline reflected, in fact, quite large final doses of bupivacaine. I think that this is within the safety limits.

Dr Scott (Edinburgh): I would like to congratulate Dr Reynolds on her excellent work. In regard to blood levels of local anaesthetics, one is just a little worried about what we call a toxic level. Dr Reynolds considers this to be 2 μg per ml for bupivacaine. Of course, there is a very wide difference with lignocaine between the levels that will give early toxicity (usually considered to be 5 μg per ml) and the level that will cause convulsions (over 10 μg per ml). Work was done in Sweden quite recently in which plain bupivacaine for epidural block was used in surgical cases in doses of about 17 ml 0·5 per cent. In quite a small series, something like 120 patients, they had one grand mal convulsion and about five people who twitched. I would have thought that that makes it rather toxic but still well within the limits of safety for continuous epidurals in labour.

Dr Reynolds (in reply): With regard to toxic levels I agree that they always look a bit near the knuckle, but if you compare the toxic levels of bupivacaine and those that are sometimes recorded with lignocaine you find that in fact the margin with lignocaine is non-existent. Indeed many people have recorded toxic symptoms with 3 μg per ml of lignocaine[2] and this is a figure which is frequently achieved by the *mean* final level of lignocaine when used in continuous epidural analgesia, and even when using large single doses[3] [4]. So that although the margin of safety looks narrow we expect local anaesthetics to make the patient sleepy (this might occur at plasma bupivacaine levels between 1·6 and 2·0 μg per ml) and I think that there is plenty of margin between this and frank convulsions.

Dr Selwyn Crawford (Birmingham): May I add my congratulations. I think that the data which you presented demand a bit more amplification and I am still worried about your showing the differences in peaks between lignocaine and bupivacaine with adrenaline. (Figure 2). With reference to Figure 3 comparing bupivacaine with and without adrenaline, surely a 20 to 40 per cent difference in peak levels of concentration is a fairly large difference in terms of proportion to the baseline level? A further point I would like to ask is: were some of these studies with reference to blood levels obtained following epidural and others with reference to those obtained with systemic administration of the agent, because you introduced quite rightly the question of plasma protein binding? Now this matter must be considered separately from that of binding of the agents in the epidural space. The question has been interestingly raised in a couple of papers[5] [6] recently, of the specifically high binding of bupivacaine by certain neuro-proteins (which might or might not be associated with myelin sheath) compared to the extent to which these proteins bind lignocaine. One further point: was the pH of the solution of bupivacaine with adrenaline the same as the pH of bupivacaine plain because that is going to have an effect on binding, isn't it?

Dr Reynolds (in reply): With regard to the relative accumulation of lignocaine and bupivacaine, you cannot compare the two blood concentration ordinates because the potencies of the two drugs are different. I therefore said that all you could do was to compare the peak levels after the first dose with those after the final dose. The average rise in peak level in the bupivacaine group was only about 1½ times the initial peak level, whereas in the lignocaine group the average rise was about 3 times. With regard to the difference in the peak levels using bupivacaine with and without adrenaline, the only statistically significant difference in this series was 20 minutes after the first dose; and thereafter, because numbers were small, there was no significant difference at individual times. However, taking the series as a whole, adrenaline undoubtedly reduces plasma level 20 minutes after all doses, but because in this series it didn't noticeably prolong the duration of action of bupivacaine there was no increased tendency to accumulate over the course of labour when adrenaline was omitted. I expected a rise at the end of labour when larger doses were necessary.

With regard to protein binding, when I said that the protein binding of bupivacaine inhibited its passage across the placenta, I was referring to plasma protein binding. I also said that bupivacaine was taken up in tissues because it is a very lipid soluble drug and certainly I think its binding within the epidural space is probably a factor of its duration of action; I don't think anybody has determined exactly what local anaesthetics are doing in that area but I imagine binding is a factor which is delaying the absorption of bupivacaine. It *is* more slowly absorbed than the other drugs that I have studied.

With regard to the pH of the solutions, I believe that the pH of bupivacaine with adrenaline is lower than that without adrenaline. I am quite prepared to believe that this might alter the binding. However, in our series this did not significantly alter the duration of action. Now some people have found that it alters the duration of action of bupivacaine marginally. It didn't in this case. Of course, it is going to inhibit absorption and there are a lot of reasons for this.

Professor Simpson (London Hospital): Dr Reynolds showed a comparison in blood concentrations of bupivacaine when given with and without adrenaline to mothers in early labour. I would like to ask if these patients were normotensive.

Dr Reynolds (in reply): Yes they were.

Professor Simpson: It is not generally appreciated that the addition of adrenaline makes no difference to the length of action of local analgesic drugs as long as the patient remains normotensive. Table 2 shows the length of action of lignocaine, prilocaine and bupivacaine each with and

Table 2

Length of Action of Local Analgesic Drugs in the Thoracic Epidural Space

		Duration to Recession of Two Segments	
Patient	Drug	With Adrenaline	Without Adrenaline
1	Lignocaine 1·5%	65	65
2	,,	60	60
3	,,	61	57
4	Prilocaine 1·5%	48	46
5	,,	48	43
6	,,	56	54
7	Bupivacaine 0·375%	122	118
8	,,	140	130
9	,,	129	126

39

without adrenaline given for thoracic epidural analgesia.[7] It can be seen that in normotensive patients the length of action of local analgesic drugs is remarkably constant and that the addition of adrenaline makes no difference to the length of action. It is in patients who become hypotensive that adrenaline may have a marked effect.

REFERENCES

1. Reynolds F and Taylor G (1970). *Maternal and neonatal blood concentrations of bupivacaine: a comparison with lignocaine during continuous extradural analgesia.* Anaesthesia, **25**, 14

2. Jewitt D E, Kishon Y and Thomas M (1968). *Lignocaine in the management of arrhythmias after acute myocardial infarction.* Lancet, **1**, 266

3. Thomas J, Climie C R, Long G and Nighjoy J E (1969). *The influence of adrenaline on the maternal plasma levels and placental transfer of lignocaine following lumbar epidural administration.* Brit. J. Anaesth. **41**, 1029

4. Braid D P and Scott D B (1965). *The systemic absorption of local analgesic drugs*, Brit. J. Anaesth. **37**, 394

5. Bromage P R and Gertel M (1970). *Evaluation of two new local anaesthetics for major conduction blockade.* Canad. Anaesth. Soc. J. **17**, 557

6. Wilkinson G R and Lund P C (1970). *Bupivacaine levels in plasma and cerebrospinal fluid following peridural administration.* Anesthesiology, **33**, 482

7. Ellis R H, Hillman G and Simpson B R J (1970). *The duration of action of local analgesic drugs in thoracic extradural analgesia.* Progress in Anesthesiology, 1241.

Epidural Analgesia and Foetal Welfare

PROFESSOR B R J SIMPSON (The London Hospital)

Abolition of pain in labour is, in itself, sufficient motive for undertaking epidural analgesia, provided that the wellbeing of the foetus is not prejudiced. However, epidural analgesia has been shown to have advantages, not only to the foetus in conditions such as cervical dystocia, prolonged labour, prematurity and post-maturity, but also for mothers suffering from a diversity of conditions, including cardiovascular disease. Foetal homeostasis depends on adequacy of both the maternal cardiovascular system and placental blood flow. Aspects of epidural analgesia likely to affect foetal welfare will therefore be discussed under the headings of:

Uterine tone and contractions;
Placental blood flow;
Direct effect of local analgesic drugs on the foetus; and
Birth canal tone.

1. *Factors affecting uterine tone and contractions*

Firstly, in 1959 Friedman and Sachtleben[1] noted that injection of fluids, including saline, into the epidural space tended to inhibit uterine contractions for some 15–20 minutes. It was postulated that this effect was due to change in the relationship between dural and epidural pressures. If so, it might be likely to be seen more frequently following caudal epidural injections where larger volumes of fluid are required.

Secondly, in 1961 Vasicka and Kretchmer[2], on the evidence of intra-amniotic pressure measurements, demonstrated that uncomplicated conduction analgesia had no effect on uterine tone. Maternal hypertension and hypotension, however, respectively increased and decreased uterine contractility. If therefore, hypotension results from epidural analgesia, uterine contractility may be decreased.

Thirdly, the addition of adrenaline to local analgesic solutions for epidural injections in obstetrics is a controversial subject because of the potential effect of adrenaline on uterine contractility. However, Bonica[3] reports that epidural injection of up to 20 ml of local analgesic solutions with a concentration of 1 : 200,000 adrenaline had no effect on uterine contracility as measured by a sensitive tocodynamometer. Furthermore, Ward and his colleagues[4] have demonstrated the advantageous effect on cardiac output of adding adrenaline to local analgesic solutions for epidural use. On the other hand, Gunther and Bauman[5] produced evidence of prolongation of the first stage of labour when solutions containing adrenaline are used. However, this conclusion should be interpreted with considerable caution since some 20% of their patients developed hypotension following epidural injection, and the prolongation of labour is more likely to have been due to maternal hypotension than to adverse effects on uterine contractility of solutions containing adrenaline.

Fourthly, in the presence of disordered uterine function, epidural analgesia enhances foetal welfare since it is a treatment of choice for this

41

condition. This aspect will be expanded by Dr Moir later in the Symposium.

2. *Factors affecting placental blood flow*

Independently of the effect of maternal hypotension on uterine contractility, maternal hypotension may adversely affect placental perfusion. Hypovolaemia, possibly due to ante-partum haemorrhage, the supine hypotensive syndrome, vascular accident or a toxic response to the local analgesic drug must be excluded before sympathetic blockade from epidural injection is accepted as the cause of maternal hypotension. Elevation of the lower limbs, elastic stockings, change of posture, and intravascular infusion are the appropriate treatments of unwanted hypotension due to sympathetic blockade. Particularly in obstetrical practice, vasopressor drugs should be used only as a last resort and after all other possible causes of foetal distress have been eliminated. Peripheral vasoconstrictor drugs such as methoxamine and phenylephrine are contra-indicated since the rise in maternal blood pressure is associated with a further decrease in uterine blood flow[6]. James and his colleagues[7] provide evidence that if maternal hypotension *must* be treated by a vasopressor, then the interests of uterine blood flow are likely to be best served by ephedrine, with mephentermine and metaraminol as second and third choices. These authors stress that even with ephedrine, correction of maternal blood pressure may be accompanied by a further reduction in uterine blood flow in some 5% of subjects.

3. *Direct effect of local analgesic drugs on the foetus*

It is now accepted that local analgesic drugs cross placental barriers to variable degrees, depending on the physicochemical properties of the drug. Gordon[8], using paracervical block, was able to correlate high foetal blood levels of local analgesic drug with foetal bradycardia, indicating a depressant effect of the drug on foetal circulation. Two points must be made: firstly, the work reported by Dr Felicity Reynolds in the previous paper supports the findings of Tucker *et al*[9] that the UV: maternal bupivacaine ratios at delivery were significantly less than the corresponding ratios for lignocaine and mepivacaine. This demonstrates an important advantage of bupivacaine over the other drugs in obstetrical practice. Secondly, although foetal blood levels of local analgesic drug are likely to be less following epidural block than those following paracervical block, foetal bradycardia due to a high level of drug is not necessarily an indication for immediate delivery—it can be differentiated from bradycardia due to foetal hypoxia by the time of onset and absence of correlation with uterine contractions. Redistribution of the drug and the greater rate of metabolism by the mother will result in passage of the drug from the foetus to the maternal circulation across the placenta. Therefore, unless the foetal condition is deteriorating, some 10–15 minutes should be allowed for this mechanism to become established.

Foetal intoxication has also been reported[10] as a result of accidental direct injection of local analgesic drug into the foetus as the result of misplaced caudal extradural needles and catheters. This catastrophe is, of course, preventable.

42

4. Factors affecting birth canal tone

An increased incidence of failure of foetal head rotation and a higher incidence of forceps delivery are usually items for discussion in relation to epidural analgesia for obstetrics. These subjects are dealt with later in the symposium and therefore do not require further expansion.

Conclusions

In summary I agree wholeheartedly with Moir and Willocks[11], who advocate that it is essential for the technique of epidural analgesia to be available in obstetrical practice when it is specially indicated. I also agree with Doughty[12], who argues that in 1970 this technique should be available in normal labour purely for social and humanitarian reasons. Nevertheless, it is only fair that one's admitted enthusiasm for relieving maternal distress should be curbed by awareness of the potential hazards to the foetus.

REFERENCES

1. Friedman E A and Sachtleben M R (1959). *Caudal anesthesia: The factors that influence its effect on labor.* Obstet. Gynec. **13,** 442

2. Vasicka A and Kretchmer H (1961). *Effects of conduction and inhalation anesthesia on uterine contractions. Experimental study of the influence of anesthesia on intra-amniotic pressures.* Amer. J. Obstet. Gynec. **82,** 600

3. Bonica J J (1969). *Comments on comparative effects of prilocaine and lidocaine during peridural anesthesia for obstetrics.* Survey of Anesthesiology, **13,** 393

4. Ward R J, Bonica J J, Freund F G, Akamatsu T, Danziger F and Engelesson S (1965). *Epidural and subarachnoid anesthesia: cardiovascular and respiratory effects.* J. Amer. med. Assoc. **191,** 275

5. Gunther R E and Bauman J (1969). *Obstetrical caudal anesthesia: 1. A randomized study comparing 1% mepivacaine with 1% lidocaine plus epinephrine.* Anesthesiology, **31,** 5

6. Greiss F C Jr and Crandell D L (1965). *Therapy for hypotension induced by spinal anesthesia during pregnancy.* J. Amer. med. Assoc., **191,** 793

7. James F M III, Greiss F C Jr and Kemp R A (1970). *An evaluation of vasopressor therapy for maternal hypotension during spinal anesthesia.* Anesthesiology, **33,** 25

8. Gordon H (1968). *Fetal bradycardia after paracervical block. Correlation with fetal and maternal blood levels of local anesthetic.* New England J. Med. **279,** 910

9. Tucker G T, Boyes R N, Bridenbaugh P O and Moore D C (1970). *Binding of anilide-type local anesthetics in human plasma.* Anesthesiology **33,** 304

10. Finster M, Poppers P J, Sinclair J C, Morishma H O and Daniel S S (1965). *Accidental intoxication of the fetus with local anesthetic drug during caudal anesthesia.* Amer. J. Obstet. Gynec. **92,** 922

11. Moir D D and Willocks J (1970). *Selective epidural analgesia and the forceps rate.* Brit. J. Anaesth. **42,** 269

12. Doughty A (1970). *Selective epidural analgesia and the forceps rate.* Brit. J. Anaesth. **42,** 269

Mr A Noble (Westminster Hospital): May I congratulate Professor Simpson on his beautifully lucid paper. I felt uneasy at one point when he discussed the treatment of hypotension with vasopressors; I wonder whether this is ever indicated in the labouring patient. I cannot recall an uncomplicated case in which the hypotension was not corrected by postural change.

Professor Simpson (in reply): I tried to point out that the use of vaso-pressors was a last resort. I agree that it is rarely necessary, but if it is necessary, then I think that the choice of vasopressor which is used is important.

Dr Hargrove (Westminster Hospital): How would you define hypotension in this context? Do you take an absolute figure, for example, 80 or 90 mm.Hg systolic or are you going to define a hypotensive episode as one in which there is a fall of 20 mm.Hg. from the pre-epidural pressure?

Professor Simpson (in reply): I do not believe in quoting absolute levels. One must take into account firstly the mother's initial blood pressure level, and secondly, which is perhaps more important, the state of the placental circulation. The degenerating placenta is obviously going to become more inadequate with a fall of maternal blood pressure than a healthy one. I am reluctant to see the maternal systolic blood pressure fall below 100 mm.Hg. without trying to take steps to remedy this.

The Chairman: May I ask Professor Simpson a question more pointedly than has been put before. Are there any circumstances in obstetrics other than an inadvertent total spinal anaesthetic in which you would advocate giving pressor drugs?

Professor Simpson (in reply): If maternal hypotension results in foetal asphyxia, as evidenced by foetal bradycardia made worse by uterine contractions, I would use conservative measures to raise the maternal blood pressure such as shifting the position of the uterus, raising the foot of the bed, using elastic stockings and increasing circulating blood volume. If these measures were not adequate and foetal distress persisted, I would use vasopressors, but only as a last resort.

Dr Hughes (Chertsey): In cases of pre-eclamptic toxaemia where there is an abnormally high systemic blood pressure could you indicate what you consider to be a reasonably safe relative fall in blood pressure with particular reference to the placental circulation.

Professor Simpson (in reply): I would not like to give a definite reply to this question. As I said before, in patients with pre-eclampsia there is a tendency towards placental insufficiency. I would watch carefully for evidence of foetal distress in association with the change in maternal blood pressure. The change of blood pressure that one would accept under these circumstances with a pre-raised blood pressure would be greater than one would normally consider desirable. I think that one has to take into account the needs of the foetus as well as those of the mother.

Mr Noble (Westminster Hospital): I am sorry to labour this point again, Professor, but may I put another view. Normally, epidural-induced hypotension with associated foetal bradycardia will return to normal after postural change. The only time I remember that this did not happen was in a patient where intra-partum placental abruption had occurred. If, after postural correction, maternal hypotension and apparent foetal distress persists, would it not be safer to deliver the baby? I am anxious lest the use of a vasopressor might cause further harm to the foetus.

Professor Simpson (in reply): I think that this is a very fair point. You may remember that ante-partum haemorrhage was on my list of possible causes of maternal hypotension.

Mr Frampton (Warwick): As an obstetrician awaiting the onset of pain relief from an epidural block I have noticed that the pain of the contractions does persist for about 10 to 20 minutes. Were you suggesting perhaps that the amplitude of the contractions was lessened or that the contractions were in fact obliterated? With regard to the problem of hypotension, do anaesthetists generally take into consideration that there is often a rise of blood pressure in normal labour in the patient who has been normotensive during pregnancy?

Professor Simpson (in reply): In answer to the first point, I think that in many patients the contractions do continue but that in others there is an inhibition of contractions for a period of 15 to 20 minutes. In answer to the second point, we do take into account the rise of blood pressure in normal labour in patients who have been normotensive during pregnancy. If you are suggesting that my trying to keep the maternal blood pressure at the level of 100 mm.Hg is being very conservative, then I will go along with the concept that I am conservative in this matter. My concern is not solely with the mother, it is also with the foetus and if the foetus is showing no evidence of distress under these circumstances, I take no action. I would like to emphasise yet again that I am advocating the use of vasopressors only as a *last resort*. If you use them as a last resort, there are some which are preferable to others. The present evidence would suggest that ephedrine and mephentermine are the drugs of choice in the unhappy situation in which you do everything else first to avoid the necessity of using them.

Dr Redmen (Guildford): I think that the probem of hypotension could be more serious if the patient having the epidural had been given pethidine and promazine an hour or two previously. It is well known that the compensatory vasoconstriction which occurs above the block may play an important part in the maintenance of normal blood pressure, and this corrective mechanism may be interfered with in such patients. For a variety of reasons we do not perform epidurals as a routine on our patients and it is not uncommon for the anaesthetist to be asked to provide epidural analgesia on patients who have been in prolonged labour and who have had one or more doses of pethidine and promazine. I remember one such case who had received pethidine 120 mg and promazine 50 mg intramuscularly 90 minutes before the epidural. Her blood pressure dropped alarmingly. As change of posture did not restore the blood pressure to an acceptable level, I had to resort to a vasopressor in this particular case. I would have thought that this was surely a clear indication for giving a vasopressor.

Prof Simpson (in reply): If you have done everything else, the things which we have already discussed, raising the feet, elastic stockings, turning them to the left, pre-loading the circulation, then I can only refer you to Mr Noble for further argument.

Mr Noble (Westminster Hospital): It is interesting that our experience, using over 1,000 epidural blocks annually is different to yours. It is possibly because most of our patients choose an epidural in the first instance and do not have intramuscular drugs as well.

Dr J Selwyn Crawford (Birmingham): Unfortunately, there is a lot of nonsense talked about hypotension as a hazard of regional block in obstetrics. It has been a hazard because the caval occlusion syndrome[1] has not been recognised or sufficiently understood in obstetric circles in North America and in this country. The whole issue has been confused by the fact that the supine hypotensive syndrome due to vena caval occlusion is more prominently observable when a patient has had an epidural block. That form of hypotension is not directly referable to autonomic blockade, which is what we should be discussing following Professor Simpson's paper.

Having excluded the group of patients who are hypotensive because of caval occlusion, one should then differentiate between two other factors which can contribute to a fall of blood pressure in a patient during labour. The one with which we are concerned specifically is an actual autonomic blockade: loss of vasomotor tone. Two other contributory factors are these: there is the patient who is having pain during labour as a result of which her blood pressure rises. When she is given relief from pain her blood pressure falls. That condition is characterised by a general slow declination in blood pressure, it isn't a sudden sharp drop 15, 20 or 30 minutes after the epidural injection has been made. The other situation is the patient who is toxaemic. We know that there are late toxaemics who begin to develop hypertension or episodes of hypertension during labour without having been within the category of defined hypertension during late pregnancy. Their blood pressure begins to rise once they go into labour. This rise can be reversed by pain relief as produced by epidural block, and that again is not referable to autonomic blockade. That is an acceptable fall of blood pressure and not one which demands to be treated. It is an acceptable response to a therapeutic measure. Surely the situation that I think that Professor Simpson is talking about is an acute fall of blood pressure due to autonomic blockade resulting from massive block of sympathetic outflow. I would support what he said, you do everything you can before you finally resort to giving a vasopressor. If nothing else is working you've got to give something which is immediately available for the sake of the mother, but, as you have said, it has to be left as a very final resort.

REFERENCE

1. Lees M M, Scott D B and Kerr M G (1970). *Haemodynamic changes associated with labour*. J. Obstet. Gynaec. Brit. Cwlth. **77**, 29

Practical Considerations Concerning the Efficacy of Epidural Analgesia in Labour

DR RONALD GREEN (St George's Hospital, London)

Of all techniques used in anaesthesia, epidural analgesia for the control of pain in labour requires the most meticulous attention to detail. For this reason I make no apologies for taking this opportunity of discussing a few practical points in technique.

Selection of Cases

There are few absolute contra-indications to the use of epidural analgesia in labour which I will discuss in a moment, but there is one contra-indication to which I would like to draw your attention particularly and that is the patients' unwillingness to be subjected to this procedure. The patient must never be actively persuaded to have this type of analgesia against her will. There are a number of psychological as well as physical reasons why a patient may be unsuitable for this procedure and these must always be respected by the anaesthetist.

Other contra-indications are:

1. Previous Caesarean section
   (a) Classical Caesarean section
   (b) Lower segment Caesarean Section accompanied by disproportion
2. Sepsis on back
3. Patient on anti-coagulant therapy
4. 'Back troubles'
5. Neurological disease   *Diabetes neuropathy*

In regard to the latter I should like to record and seek an opinion on a specific case.

A patient of 21 years of age was very keen to have a painless labour for her first baby, but at the age of 12 years had had severe meningitis which had left no neurological sequelae. The obstetrician wondered whether I would be prepared to do an epidural for her. After careful consideration I could not see that there was any logical contra-indication and agreed to do it when the time came. I would like to hear if anyone has any strong views about this decision.

Although the block was ultimately fully successful, I was somewhat disconcerted by the fact that each top-up took a full 25 minutes to become effective and lasted for only 90 minutes. I therefore could not wait for the return of sensation before adding more local anaesthetic which had to be given well in advance of the expected return of sensation.

Timing of the Block

I still consider it unwise to inject the local anaesthetic into the epidural space until the patient is in established labour. My reason for this is mainly because the block may delay the onset of labour, but also if the patient is allowed to feel a few strong contractions she has a greater appreciation of what is being done for her, as well as a feeling that she has contributed something to her child's birth.

However, because of staff shortages we have often inserted the catheter at any time after the onset of 'early' labour to suit the anaesthetists' convenience, provided that the patient has decided by this time that she would like to have an epidural. Alternatively, if it is intended to rupture the membranes under diazepam or light general anaesthesia the opportunity may be taken to insert the catheter and this saves the stress of the procedure during established labour. If an epidural block is used for the amniotomy itself, then I prefer to give no further top-up until labour has been established. I would be interested to know if anyone would disagree with this practice on the grounds that exceptionally no analgesia is necessary in the ensuing labour. To support this point I should like to quote the following case:

I was asked to see a primigravida who claimed to have a very low threshold of pain and requested an epidural for her labour. Her membranes had ruptured and she appeared to be in early labour; I placed a catheter into the epidural space but injected no local. I left my telephone number so that the midwife could call me when labour was established and pain relief was required. I was called six hours later with the head on the perineum. She had hardly been aware that labour had commenced. I am ashamed to admit that I took full credit for the painless labour!

Site of Epidural Puncture

A point that has already been mentioned is the question of where in the lumbar region the epidural puncture should be done. I tend to teach the residents to puncture at L2-3 or L3-4, because at this level the risk of cord damage is minimal. I do not allow them to puncture any higher until I am quite confident that they have the feel of the ligaments and know exactly where they are during the passage of the needle. This is usually after they have performed at least 20 blocks—some may require to perform as many as 50.

For those with experience some advantage is to be gained by a high puncture at T12–L1. In this space with the catheter no further than one inch within the epidural space to avoid wandering of the catheter tip, minimal doses can be used for the first stage of labour, 3–5 ml often being sufficient. These doses produce no change in blood pressure or weakness of the legs, in fact no subjective symptoms of a block whatsoever. There is the disadvantage, however, that it becomes more difficult to anaesthetise the perineum for the second stage of labour. Frequently 10–15 ml of lignocaine with the patient in a steep head-up tip for 10–15 minutes has been required to anaesthetise the sacral roots.

One small point upon which I would like to ask advice concerns the fixation of the syringe during the labour. I have for a number of years used plastic syringes for obstetric epidurals as I find these are much easier to handle than glass ones, but I run frequently into the problem of the syringe nozzle breaking off when the mother moves around. It would be useful if anyone has any hints on how to prevent this. Strapping the syringe to the right leg has solved the problem to some extent.

Sterile Precautions

Apart from ensuring that the correct solution is used, strict asepsis is probably the most important discipline in this technique.

The use of the Millipore bacterial filter is, I believe, the most important safeguard in this respect. The efficiency of this device will, however, depend upon the filter being intact. It is therefore prudent that these filters, which have been assembled by experts, should be used once only. Attempts to change the filter and re-sterilise should perhaps be resisted, unless skilled staff is available. I have allowed re-sterilisation of filters in gynaecological cases for some time, but have not infrequently found the filters damaged. The temperature and pressure of sterilisation is critical—modern autoclaves operate at a temperature and pressure which is too high for this purpose. Gamma-Ray sterilisation is perhaps the method of choice.

As an additional precaution to the filter I like to enclose both the filter and syringe in a plastic sleeve—a disposable plastic glove with the tip of one finger cut off is a useful alternative. Does everyone agree that these measures are adequate—or is it considered necessary to scrub up for each syringe change?

Top-Up Routine

There is no single factor more important to the success of a labour epidural, so far as the mother is concerned, than topping up at the correct time. This raises the thorny point of who should give the top-up doses. The question of allowing midwives to do this has been discussed on many occasions. I believe that, provided the necessary training is given and precautions are taken, the midwives can perform this very valuable service when medical staff are not readily available, as they can ensure that there is no delay between the return of sensation and the reintroduction of the block. At St George's Hospital it has now been agreed that senior midwives should be allowed to give the top-up doses subject to the following provisions:

1. They are certified as having attended special tuition on this technique.
2. That the first top-up through the catheter, which must be done by an anaesthetist, has presented no problems.
3. That the exact dose to be given be recorded by the anaesthetist, and the syringe containing the drug attached to the catheter.
4. That the anaesthetist should be contacted by telephone immediately prior to the top-up for final instructions.
5. That careful attention to the bladder should be given before each top-up. The patient is urged to pass water before each top-up. If they are unable to do so, and the bladder is 'full', then a catheter is passed.

The safety of this procedure must depend upon the belief that the catheter, once in situ, will not shift its position. If there is any firm evidence that this is not so, then this practice cannot be regarded as safe. It would be most valuable to hear from anyone who has had complications following top-up doses, *e.g.* hypotension or unusual spread, when the previous epidural injections with the same quantity of local have been uncomplicated.

Management of the Partially Effective Block

For various reasons the initial block may not be completely effective. The underlying causes for this are sometimes obscure and difficult to correct, but usually some alteration in posture or position of the catheter will do the trick.

The most difficult condition to correct is a completely unilateral block. I have seen this twice and on both occasions I have had to revert to conventional analgesia. I believe that the failure of the block to spread is due to an epidural septum and that apart from inserting a second catheter on the other side no manipulation of the catheter or posturing the patient will make any difference. It is important to give these patients analgesics while trying to achieve a more effective block.

The most common failure is persistent pain in the groin during contractions, this is most likely to occur if the initial dose is given while the patient is still lying on her side. It can usually be corrected by giving a further dose with the patient lying on the opposite side.

Complete failure to achieve any analgesia is rare in experienced hands, and is usually due to the catheter ending up in a paravertebral space. I believe that the commonest fault here is the temptation to thread too much of the catheter into the space. I always pull the catheter out after insertion so that the 10 cm mark is at skin level, and since doing this I have not encountered this trouble.

Failure to get adequate analgesia for the second stage of labour may occur if a high puncture is used and small doses of local anaesthetic are given. It is important that the sacral roots should be blocked as soon as full dilatation has occurred. I usually use 10–12 ml of local anaesthetic with a steep head up tip, or with the patient sitting up. If this stage of labour is likely to be short, as in multiparae, it may be an advantage to use lignocaine rather than bupivacaine.

It is important that the patient should not be allowed to suffer due to partial failure of the block, and therefore analgesics must not be withheld, but except for the rare event of the totally unilateral block, I have found this seldom necessary provided that the top-up doses are given at the correct time.

DISCUSSION

The Chairman: Dr Green has given us many points for discussion the most controversial of which may be the practice of allowing the top-ups to be done by midwives. I think that this is the key to the wider use of epidural analgesia in labour.

Dr Rubin (Charing Cross Hospital): With regard to the safety of top-ups by midwives, Moore has reported the apparent perforation of the dura by the catheter after a first or even a second satisfactory response to the injection of local analgesic[1]. He suggested that the pulsations of the dura mater against the catheter tip could result in the weakening of the dura and the catheter eroding into the subarachnoid space. I have personally seen this complication in the United States, although the epidural catheters that we were using had cut-off sharp tips and were more rigid than the round ended Portex variety in general use in this country.

I feel that the problem of fixing a syringe to the patient can be overcome by the use of the Tuohy-Borst Adaptor made by Becton-Dickinson & Co. (see page 93). With this Luer-fitting adaptor, which has a sterile cap, there is no need to attach the syringe except during the injection of local analgesic and there is no risk of contamination between injections.

Dr J Selwyn Crawford (Birmingham): With respect to the use of the Millipore filter I do not accept that it is necessary to throw it away after use. We have now given over 1,200 epidurals in the last eighteen months and started off with a stock of 2 or 3 dozen filters. We have not added to that stock. These filters have been re-tested bacteriologically and have been pronounced satisfactory. Inexperienced personnel are not allowed to change the filter disc. It is changed either by the Superintendent Midwife or by the Theatre Sister and the Millipore filter is then re-autoclaved. We check the filter disc each time before the filter is attached to the catheter. I have not the slightest doubt as to the efficiency of this system and I see no reason why the filters should be thrown away after being used but once.

We leave the filter open during the course of labour. For the top-up injections we merely fill up a syringe and plug it on to the end of the filter. The problem of the filter being obstructed by the broken syringe nozzle does not arise as I do not understand the need for some sort of plug at the end of the Millipore filter. I doubt whether the plug is likely to be of any greater hygienic benefit than is the filter itself.

Dr Green mentioned that neurological disease in the patient might contra-indicate the use of epidural analgesia. I think that, in general, these are more medico-legal than specifically medical contra-indications. Our policy has been based on a reading of the literature, our own discussions and, I hope, on a certain amount of common sense. We do not consider that a history of meningitis or poliomyelitis contra-indicates an epidural. We do not consider that epilepsy, psychiatric disorders or migraine are contra-indications. We do consider that epidural analgesia is contra-indicated in patients with disc lesions or lumbo-sciatic pain. There is a doubt about diabetic neuropathy because that might continue to develop during the subsequent twelve months and if the patient develops a foot-drop she is liable to blame the epidural and not think about the effect of the diabetes. Certainly cerebrovascular disorder, either haemorrhage or aneurysm, is not a contra-indication but rather an indication for a lumbar epidural block. A history of intracranial tumour is an indication for a caudal block but not a lumbar epidural because of the danger of a dural puncture in a patient with raised intracranial pressure.

In summary then, our attitude with regard to neurological disease and the use of epidural analgesia is determined more by the possibility of litigation rather than by any specific medical contra-indication.

Dr Hargrove (Westminster Hospital): Firstly, I would like to challenge Dr Crawford's statement about the Millipore filters. The fact that the bacteriologist has examined, say, 12 successive filters after autoclaving and found them to be competent does not mean to say that the 13th one is not going to be faulty. We started off by changing the filter disc and autoclaving after each case. To my consternation when I opened two of the filters at random, I found that the filter disc had become brittle and shattered. We no longer continue this practice and considering that the cost of the whole Millipore filter is about 41 pence we do not regard this as highly expensive, particularly when compared with the cost of other things in the Health Service.

Secondly, we do not leave the needle on the catheter. We cut off the Luer fitting at the end of the catheter, attach an ordinary ureteric catheter chuck (obtainable from Down Bros.) to this cut end and connect the Millipore filter to the chuck. A rubber cap is then placed over the open end of the filter.

Lastly, regarding midwives: right from the very beginning of the epidural service at Westminster Hospital, we decided that it would be impossible to carry on the service without midwife co-operation. Initially, there was slight opposition because they thought it would involve them in a great deal more work. Now, they are totally converted and, in fact, they make the request for the patients to have epidurals more and more frequently. In order that the midwives should be allowed to top-up the epidurals we had to go through the nursing administration and the General Nursing Council to obtain the necessary permission, but we have no problems at all now. Of course, an anaesthetist always gives the first dose of local analgesic.

The Chairman: Dr Hargrove, may I ask you to comment very shortly on Dr Green's opinion that the mother should experience a little pain before you give the epidural. I believe that at Westminster Hospital you put in the catheter before the contractions begin.

Dr Hargrove: Yes, we are quite content to put the catheter in right at the beginning of labour or at induction. I do not think that any of us would give the first dose of local anaesthetic until the woman was in established labour so that all our patients feel some discomfort at the start of labour. We do not wait until the patient has reached 4–5 cm dilatation, or even full dilatation, before giving any analgesic as happens in some centres in America. As soon as the patient has discomfort and regular contractions, I think this is the time to institute analgesia.

Dr Chatterjee (Birmingham): I would like to ask Dr Green what is his experience regarding the use of epidural analgesia in the conduct of breech deliveries.

Dr Green (in reply): Breech deliveries are not common. We have done one or two epidurals for breech deliveries and found nothing to contra-indicate them. Epidural analgesia seems to be a very good technique, it allows the slow removal of the head providing you have got good perineal analgesia and I do not think that there is anything special to say about it.

Dr Fraser-Jones (Solihull): At the Maternity Unit based upon Solihull Hospital we have undertaken ten breech deliveries under epidural block and it is my opinion that this is the method of choice for breech delivery. Two of the breeches delivered spontaneously, one by breech extraction and the remainder were assisted breech deliveries. The one case of breech extraction was easily performed.

Considerable discussion has taken place between myself and the obstetricians regarding breech delivery under epidural analgesia and it is agreed that careful assessment of the case is essential prior to undertaking the block. The obstetricians believe that in the case of a large breech baby it is better not to attempt vaginal delivery and that they would hold the same point of view if there was any degree of pelvic disproportion. Quite obviously a mis-assessment can be made but it has been our experience, so far, that epidural block is exceptionally suitable for breech delivery and is far better than the instantaneous general anaesthesia that some obstetricians used to demand.

Mr Pearson (Birmingham): I would like to make what I consider to be a most important point in regard to the use of epidural analgesia during breech delivery.

To achieve optimum results in the conduct of a breech delivery, the aim should be to deliver with minimal interference. To this end, the importance of retaining effective maternal effort cannot be overstressed. We have shown in Birmingham that whether or not the urge to push is maintained there is an increase in the overall duration of the second stage in cephalic presentation due, we think, to an impairment of the mother's ability to push. Thus it seems likely that the use of epidural analgesia may pre-dispose to a number of unneceessary breech extractions and other manoeuvres which would be likely to increase perinatal mortality. For this reason we have tended not to use this form of analgesia when the breech is presenting.

REFERENCE

Moore D C (1969). *Regional Block* 4th Edition, p467 Chas. C Thomas, Springfield, Illinois

Complications of Epidural Analgesia

(a) Neurological Complications

DR J EDMONDS (University College Hospital, London)

Introduction

An epidural injection is the most certain and effective way of producing pain relief in labour, and it is being used by anaesthetists with increasing frequency. The publication of case reports describing neurological damage following epidural injections may well deter many anaesthetists from practising the method. The following case report may appear to give some substance to these fears. It is hoped that the discussion will put them into perspective.

Case Report

A fit 24 year old woman was admitted in early labour. She had previously had a vaginal delivery of a full term normal infant and there was no history of neurological nor musculo-skeletal illness. Eight hours after admission her labour was progressing slowly and, as she was in considerable distress, it was decided to give her an epidural injection.

With the patient in the left lateral position, the lumbar skin area was cleaned with iodine, followed by chlorhexidine in spirit; a Tuohy needle was inserted into the epidural space at the L3-4 interspace using loss of resistance to air as an indicator. A Portex catheter was passed in a cephalad direction for 4 cms and during this procedure the patient made no complaints of pain nor parasthesia. A test dose of 2 ml bupivacaine 0·5% with 1 : 200,000 adrenaline injected through a Millipore filter produced no symptoms, and a further 5 ml of this solution was given.

This gave her considerable relief, although she still had slight pain in her left groin during contractions. A further 8 ml bupivacaine with adrenaline was given through the catheter after 2½ hours, and 1 hour later she was delivered vaginally without the use of forceps. Five hours after insertion, the epidural catheter was removed and the tip was seen to be clean and intact. Regular recordings showed that her blood pressure never fell below 120/70 during the procedure.

After delivery and while still under the effects of epidural analgesia, she had no motor power in her legs with sensory loss from L1 to S5. Forty-eight hours later she was still complaining of numbness in her back and legs. On examination she could walk, but there was a weakness on dorsiflexion of her right ankle and a loss of sensation to pinprick over the whole area of both legs below the knees. This loss of sensation did not follow a dermatome pattern but was of a stocking type of anaesthesia. Now, eighteen months later, she still complains of a feeling of 'numbness and clumsiness' in her right foot, although she walks normally without foot-drop and neurological examination shows her reflexes to be equal on the two sides.

Discussion

In assessing the cause of neurological damage following the use of an epidural injection during labour, it is necessary to differentiate between epidural causes and obstetric causes.

A. Epidural Causes of Neurological Damage

1. Direct Needle Damage

Although this is unlikely in this reported case history, the literature has three cases of damage from this cause. Bonica[1] (1957) reported one patient who had unilateral hypoalgesia on the right leg three years after the insertion of a needle at the level of the 8th thoracic segment, and a second case who had paraesthesia and pain for 5 days following introduction of a needle during a cervical epidural. Both patients complained of pain and paraesthesia during the injection. More relevant to obstetric epidurals, Birkhahn and Heifetz[2] (1961) considered that the damage giving rise to hypoalgesia and hypoesthesia on the external surface of the thigh in their patient was due to direct damage to the 2nd lumbar root following insertion of an epidural catheter. No pain was elicited during the insertion as lignocaine had already been introduced into the space.

2. Contamination

No case of epidural abscess following epidural puncture appears in the literature, but the possibility is always present. Two cases of arachnoiditis appear, one leading to a crippled patient with impaired sphincter section (Braham and Saia[3], 1958) but whether this was due to contamination or to a reaction following the injection is in doubt.

3. Accidental Spinal

This complication, with a precipitate fall in the blood pressure and dilatation of the pupils following rapidly on the injection, should not result in neurological damage if treatment is instituted rapidly and correctly.

4. Disc Prolapse

Any patient with symptoms of neurological change in the lower limbs should be suspected of having a disc lesion, even those cases appearing after an epidural injection. Lund[4] (1966) describes a fracture of a vertebral lamina following epidural puncture that led to signs of compression of the cord.

5. Haematoma

Two cases of epidural haematoma after needle insertion have been described[5] [6]. Both these cases had received anticoagulants, one before epidural puncture, and the other was started on anticoagulants with an epidural catheter in position. Symptoms of compression led to surgical evacuation of an epidural haematoma. There are no reports of epidural haematoma with patients not on anticoagulants.

6. Interference with the Blood Supply

Although the anatomical descriptions of the blood supply to the spinal cord describe many radicular arteries arising from the aorta to form a rich anastomosis with the three longitudinal spinal arteries, there appear to be many areas where the blood supply is precarious. Occlusion or diminished

flow through the spinal arteries, particularly in patients with poor flow from the aorta due to arteriosclerosis, can cause ischaemia of the cord [7].
The literature has two cases of post mortem appearances of the cord showing spinal artery insufficiency that gave rise to neurological deficits [7] [8]. It is postulated that hypotension from the epidural and the presence of adrenaline in the injected solution may cause ischaemia at this site.

7. Toxic Effects of the Injected Solution

Bromage [9] reports that patients occasionally complain of pain during the injection of bupivacaine with adrenaline as supplied in pre-mixed ampoules, and that the pH of these solutions is between 2·6 and 3·5. Bupivacaine mixed freshly with an adrenaline solution has a pH of 6·1 and does not produce pain when injected into the epidural space. Bupivacaine with adrenaline solution, when injected into muscle of a rat's leg, causes changes in that muscle compatible with denervation. Other local anaesthetics used as controls do not produce this change [10].

Table 1
Neurological Complications following Epidural Block (Massey Dawkins, 1969)

	No. of cases in series	No. of times Complication arose	
Headache	3,637	25	0·7%
Accidental Spinal	48,297	102	0·2%
Massive Extradural	16,644	28	0·1%
Transient Paralysis	32,718	48	0·1%
Permanent Paralysis	32,718	7	0·02%

In spite of these many possibilities of inflicting damage, the number of cases in the literature are relatively small. Table 1 shows some of the figures that Massey Dawkins (1969) produced following his extensive survey of the world literature [11]. Massive extradurals which are included in this list should not result in neurological sequelae if proper resuscitation is carried out. These figures may be misleadingly low. The writer knows of one death following a massive epidural and has been informed of two cases of paralysis, one permanent and one transitory, following epidurals that do not appear in the literature. Are there many other cases occurring that are not reported?

B. Obstetric Causes of Neurological Damage

There are several well recognised complications of labour and vaginal delivery that can give rise to neurological damage of the lower limbs in the absence of epidural injections, including subarachnoid haemorrhages and

Table 2
Neurological Complications following Vaginal Deliveries

Cole 1946	7 Cases	in a series of 45,000
O'Connell 1958	8 Cases	of prolapsed disc during labour
Hill 1962	5 Cases	
Moir & Myerscough 1971	6 Cases	of foot drop

exacerbation of spinal tumours. Table 2 shows the cases reported of neurological damage following vaginal deliveries in the absence of epidural anaesthesia. Cole [12], O'Connell [13] and Hill [14] report relatively serious neurological complications lasting for months, some of which were permanent. The cases in Chassar Moir's [15] series cleared in 6-8 weeks. In a survey of the literature reported in 1949, Chalmers [16] found 142 cases of lower limb neurological damage following vaginal deliveries without the use of epidural analgesia. The Obstetric Unit where the writer practises sees 150 cases delivered each month and each year there are two or three cases of foot-drop or other neurological sequelae in patients who have not received epidural analgesia. This damage was previously thought to be due to trauma within the pelvis, but many are now considered to be due to disc lesions occurring during labour. Damage to the lateral popliteal nerve from placing patients' legs in obstetric stirrups is already a recognised hazard of normal deliveries, and is likely to occur in patients receiving epidural analgesia as these patients make no complaint of pain nor discomfort at the time.

Summary and Conclusions

The cause of neurological damage following the use of epidurals in obstetrics is difficult to determine. Previous reports show that damage can occur from the epidural injection itself, but most of these cases are in a group of patients older than that normally associated with obstetrics, and several had other predisposing causes of neurological damage. It has been shown that trauma to nerve roots, both within the pelvis and from spinal disc lesions, can occur during vaginal deliveries; the subsequent assessment of the cause of neurological damage is made more difficult by the fact that the epidural analgesia itself masks the pain which goes unrecognised until the analgesia has waned.

While this method of pain relief remains under suspicion, some cases of neurological damage following epidural analgesia in obstetrics may unjustifiably be ascribed to it.

Acknowledgements

Thanks are due to Mr J M Holmes, MB BS, FRCOG, for permission to publish details of this case, and to Dr L Kaufman, MD, FFARCS, for help in preparing the manuscript.

REFERENCES

1. Bonica J J (1957). *Peridural Block: Analysis of 3,637 Cases.* Anesthesiology, **18**, 723

2. Birkhahn H J and Heifetz M (1961). *A complication following Epidural Anesthesia.* Curr. Res. Anesth. **40**, 650

3. Braham J and Saia A (1958). *Neurological Complications of epidural anaesthesia.* Brit. med. J. **ii**, 657

4. Lund P C (1960). *Peridural Analgesia and Anesthesia.* p.287. Charles C. Thomas, Illinois

5. Frumin M J and Schwartz H (1952). *Continuous Segmental Peridural Anesthesia.* Anesthesiology, **13**, 488

6. Gingrich T F (1968). *Spinal epidural haematoma following continuous epidural anesthesia.* Anesthesiology, **29**, 162

7. Davies A, Solomon B and Levene A (1958). *Paraplegia following epidural anaesthesia.* Brit. med. J. **ii**, 654

8. Urquhart-Hay D (1969). *Paraplegia following epidural anaesthesia.* Anaesthesia, **24**, 461

9. Bromage P R (1969). *An evaluation of bupivacaine in epidural analgesia for obstetrics*. Canad. Anaes. Soc. J. **16**, 46

10. Libelius R, Sonesson B, Stamenovic B A and Thesleff S (1970). *Denervation-like changes in skeletal muscle after treatment with a local anaesthetic*. Journal of Anatomy. (Lond.), **106**, 297

11. Dawkins C J M (1969). *An analysis of the complications of extradural and caudal block*. Anaesthesia, **24**, 554

12. Cole, J. T. (1946). *Maternal Obstetric Paralysis*. Amer. J. Obstet. Gynec. **52**, 372

13. O'Connell J E A (1944). *Maternal Obstetrical Paralysis*. Surg. Gynec. Obstet. **79**, 374

14. Hill E C (1962). *Maternal Obstetric Paralysis*. Amer. J. Obstet. Gynec. **83**, 1452

15. Moir J C and Myerscough P R (1971). *Munro Kerr's Operative Obstetrics*. 8th edition, p.923 Bailliere, Tindall and Cassell, London.

16. Chalmers J A (1949). *Traumatic Neuritis of the Puerperium* J. Obstet. Gynec. Brit. Emp. **56**, 205

DISCUSSION

Dr Rubin (Charing Cross Hospital): It is often said that epidural block tends to affect bladder function so that the patient may suffer post-partum retention of urine. I would like to ask Dr Edmonds if he has any views on this. I can quote the unfortunate experience of an Anaesthetic Senior Registrar who herself had an epidural for delivery which was followed by complete atony of the bladder necessitating an indwelling catheter for a period of ten days. In the end normal function resumed after the administration of neostigmine and there were no further sequelae.

Dr Edmonds (in reply): The incidence of bladder complications in non-obstetric practice is, in my experience, very low, and the literature has only one case of permanent sphincter disturbance.

In obstetric practice there is a significant incidence of bladder complications without the use of epidurals; and I can cite the case of an anaesthetic registrar who was requested to give an epidural to a patient in labour, but the patient delivered before the injection was inserted. This patient had sphincter disturbance of her bladder for 48 hours, which would have been ascribed to the epidural injection had it been given. This underlines the difficulty in assessment of the causes of this type of disturbance.

Complications of Epidural Analgesia

(b) Inferior Vena Caval Occlusion during Epidural Block

DR D B SCOTT (Royal Infirmary, Edinburgh)

The incidence of inferior vena caval occlusion in the later weeks of pregnancy is extremely high and probably is the rule rather than the exception. The effects of this occlusion, generally speaking, are unnoticed by ordinary clinical examination because the venous return is maintained through a collateral circulation and even when this is deficient, the body increases the peripheral resistance to maintain a normal blood pressure.

Figure 2

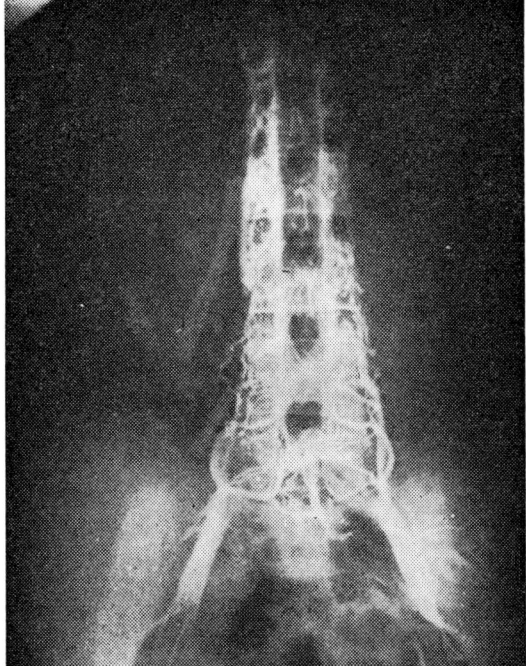

Inferior vena cavagram in supine position immediately prior to Caesarean section.

Figure 1 shows an inferior vena cavagram just prior to Caesarean section. Dye has been injected into both femoral veins and the inferior vena cava does not show up at all. This was a normal woman coming to section with no supine hypotension and you will see that the collateral circulation was being maintained mainly through the paravertebral veins and the azygos system.

Figure 2

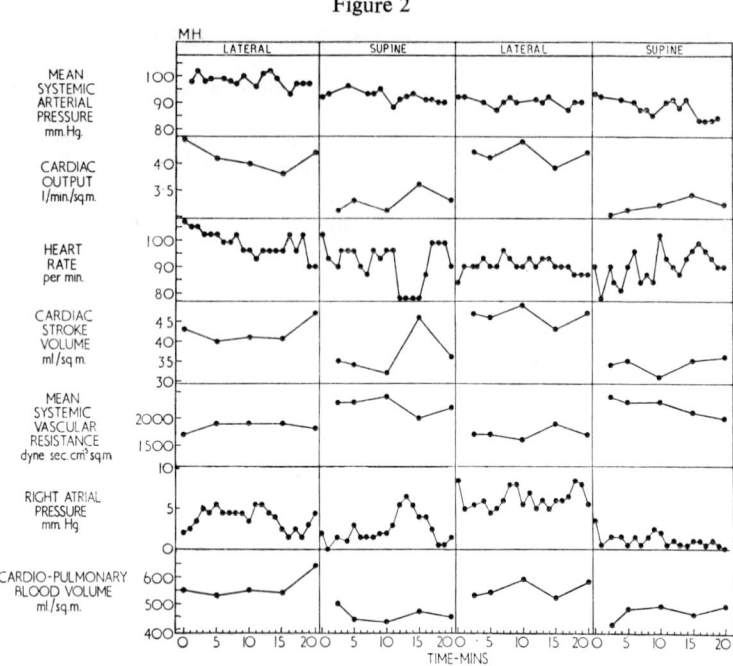

Haemodynamic changes in pregnancy associated with changes of posture from the lateral to the supine position.

Figure 2 shows what happens to the haemodynamics in these patients when they change from the lateral to the supine position. There is very little change in blood pressure with posture, but a marked fall in cardiac output each time the patient goes on to her back and to maintain normal pressure the vascular resistance is increased. We tend to talk rather loosely about blood pressure and I just want to remind you of the formula: Mean Arterial blood pressure = Cardiac Output x Peripheral Resistance. Of these three parameters the cardiac output is by far the most important. Now, it requires quite a large fall of cardiac output by itself to reduce blood pressure because the peripheral resistance increases in the intact person, and quite frequently a 25% fall in cardiac output can occur without a fall in mean arterial pressure. Therefore, a normal blood pressure cannot be equated with a normal circulation. In most women, lying supine during the later weeks of pregnancy causes a fall in cardiac output and a raised peripheral resistance. If you do anything which reduces peripheral resistance then it is quite likely that a sharp fall in blood pressure will occur and this is what I believe happens with epidural block. Supine hypotension occurs in only about 2 per cent of all pregnant women but we know that, even with very low epidural blocks up to the height of T_{10} which only affect a small proportion of the sympathetic outflow, the incidence according to Moir and Willocks[1] is around 20 % if the patients are kept in the supine position. This increased incidence of patients who become hypotensive once epidural block is given is, I think, due to the pre-existing reduction in cardiac output being shown up because they are no longer able to maintain a high vascular resistance.

Figure 3

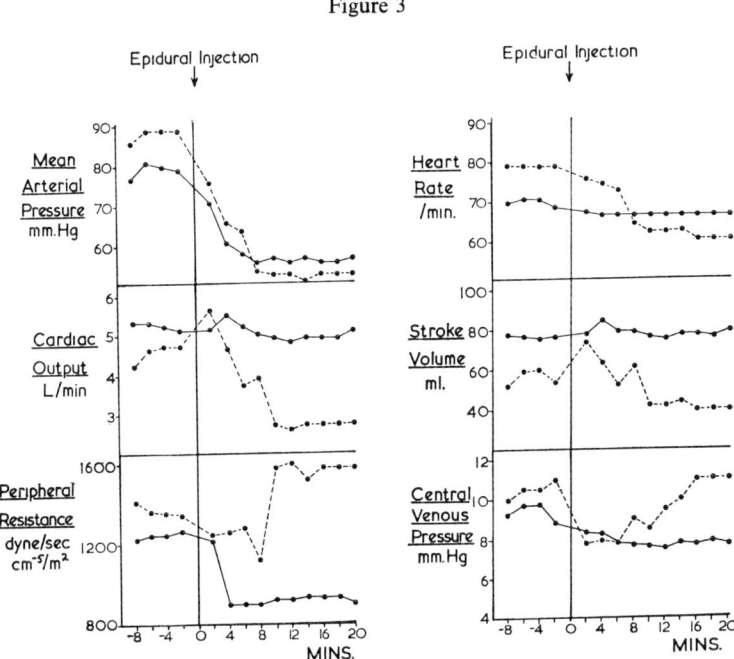

Haemodynamic effect of epidural analgesia *not* related to pregnancy.

Epidural block, unrelated to pregnancy, causes a fall in peripheral resistance but if the mean arterial pressure falls it can do so without any effect on cardiac output or heart rate (Figure 3). The dotted line is that of a single patient out of six studied who did, in fact, get a fall in cardiac output. She was the only one who dropped her heart rate, and this was probably due to a very high block up into the upper thoracic region affecting the cardiac accelerator nerves. Therefore, epidural block by itself, unless it is very high, is unlikely to have much effect on the cardiac output itself. Serious difficulties, however, do arise during epidurals in late pregnancy because the patients already have low cardiac outputs and the whole situation is made much worse because peripheral resistance is affected. Apart from inferior vena caval occlusion, a fall in cardiac output can occur if the patient develops bradycardia. I have mentioned that this may result from a very high block, but it can also occur as a result of a vaso-vagal attack.

Figure 4

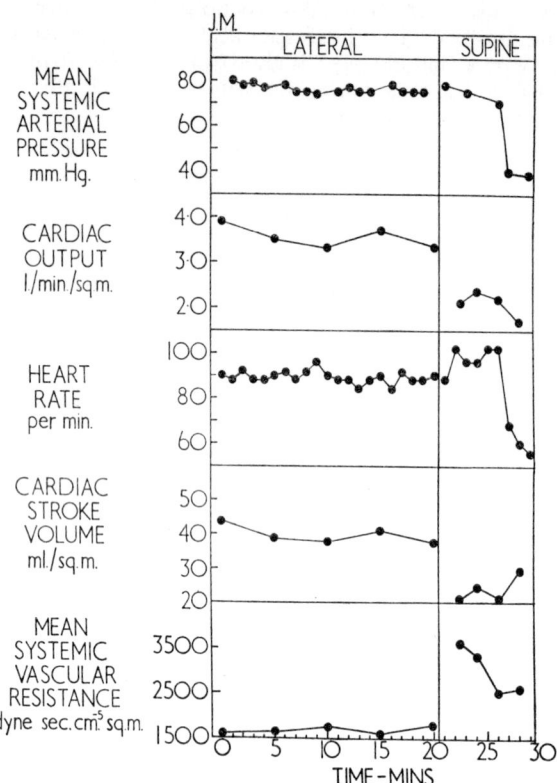

Supine hypotension in a pregnant patient *not* given an epidural.

Figure 4 shows the typical picture of supine hypotension in the non-epiduralised patient. As soon as the patient becomes supine there is a marked fall in cardiac output, but blood pressure is maintained for some two to three minutes at which point the heart rate drops sharply and then the blood pressure falls. The vascular resistance which was being maintained at high levels falls away due to the vaso-vagal attack. This is a typical faint, and supine hypotension in normal un-epiduralised patients is due to a vaso-vagal attack triggered off by the fall in cardiac output.

The treatment of hypotension following epidural block has been discussed already. Every effort should be made to eliminate the caval occlusion by posture. One problem arises when the patient has supine hypotension before the epidural block is induced. It is important to be quite sure this can be corrected by posture before undertaking the block. If hypotension develops after the block, the patient should be turned on her side and postured in such a way as to alleviate the caval occlusion. Vasopressors should only be given as a last resort, that is when hypotension of a serious nature persists in the lateral position. (The possibility that the patient is having a vaso-vagal attack should be borne in mind and the pulse rate checked.) In these circumstances I would certainly agree that ephedrine is the agent of choice because it has alpha- and beta-adrenergic stimulating properties so that both arterial pressure and cardiac output will increase. This is not the case with the alpha stimulators which tend merely to raise the blood pressure and have little effect on cardiac output.

One last word of warning; there was a maternal tragedy in Edinburgh, which I reported at the last meeting of this Society, due to caval occlusion occurring in the lateral position while the patient was bent up in the lumber puncture position. There was a long delay in inserting the catheter after an initial injection of lignocaine and the patient collapsed while lying on her side. It is quite feasible that, in this position, with the knees drawn up in front of the abdomen, the vena cava can be occluded.

REFERENCE

1. Moir D D and Willocks J (1968). *Epidural Analgesia in British Obstetrics*, Brit. J. Anaesth. **40**, 129

Complications of Epidural Analgesia

(c) Precautions against Complications

DR M E TUNSTALL (Aberdeen)

The intrinsic importance of preventing complications of epidural analgesia is amplified by the fact that good obstetrics—and that implies low maternal and perinatal morbidity and mortality—can be provided without the use of epidural analgesia. This should induce in us a sense of extra responsibility towards our patients when we administer epidurals.

I propose to give a list of essentials aimed at preventing the complications of epidural analgesia.

I believe it would be difficult to justify an 'epidural service' as distinct from the occasional 'one-off' epidural provided by a skilled anaesthetist taking total responsibility unless most of the following list of essentials can be implemented. This contains some factors which are absolutely necessary and some which are relatively so.

The absolutely essential factors in the prevention and treatment of complications of epidural analgesia are as follows:

1. Technical ability of the operator or of his direct supervisor and instructor.

2. (a) Personnel and equipment for treating complications in continuous close proximity to the patient;

(b) An intravenous cannula indwelling in the patient.

3. Sterility of equipment, technique and puncture site.

These three factors can be summed up as ability, resuscitation and sterility.

The following factors are relatively essential and partly an amplification of what has already been said.

1. That the operator is an anaesthetist. This is because in the same person you have resuscitation ability. If the labour ward has 24-hour resident cover of personnel capable of major resuscitation involving endotracheal intubation, then presumably it would be in order for obstetricians to undertake lumbar epidurals.

2. The anaesthetist should be obstetric-orientated, involved in daily labour ward activity and capable of making a proper evaluation of the mother, foetus and obstetrical situation in conjunction with his obstetrician colleagues.

3. Continuous supervision of the patient by a state registered nurse who understands the importance of relieving caval compression in obstetrical patients.

4. Frequent estimations of blood pressure and pulse for 30 minutes after each injection of local anaesthetic. A total spinal has been reported following the 3rd or 4th injection via an indwelling catheter[1].

5. All injections of local analgesic, including the test dose, should be given via an indwelling plastic cannula.

6. All punctures should be below the level of the 2nd lumbar vertebra.

7. A paramedian oblique approach is used to avoid damaging the interspinous ligament.

8. The test dose, that is the first dose, should be with lignocaine 1% without adrenaline so that, should it be an accidental intrathecal injection, one will not be injecting adrenaline into the subarachnoid space and one will not have to be responsible for a totally anaesthetised patient for so long.

9. The patient should be awake during puncture. The conscious patient is able to tell you if you are ploughing the needle through nervous tissue.

10. If a forceps delivery is required the segmental lumbar epidural should be supplemented by a pudendal and perineal block. This policy has worked very well in the Aberdeen Maternity Hospital. It saves the inconvenience of calling the epidural operator, sitting the patient up and giving a relatively large dose of solution into the epidural space with an increased risk due to extension of vasomotor block. If Caesarean section is required we normally give a standard general anaesthetic.

11. Patients under epidural analgesia should be treated as high risk cases. They should have either no food or drink, or a restricted diet of the type suggested by Crawford[2]. In the Aberdeen Maternity Hospital all patients in labour are given magnesium trisilicate mixture every two hours.

12. The woman in labour under epidural analgesia should lie on a special obstetric bed capable of being tilted head down very rapidly. A syringe, needle and ephedrine ampoules are placed on her bedside locker so that any emergency injection may be given through the indwelling intravenous cannula. Beside her should be a bag and mask resuscitation unit connected to the wall oxygen supply.

13. There are a number of contra-indications, absolute or relative, to epidural analgesia in labour, such as scarred uterus, long standing hypertension, anti-coagulant therapy and neurological disease. Furthermore, it is wise to avoid adrenaline in hyperthyroidism, mitral stenosis, severe anaemia and arterial disease. These considerations come within the orbit of common sense and physicianly knowledge.

Sterile Precautions

The Aberdeen Maternity Hospital epidural pack contains everything that may be required except the operator's gloves and the local anaesthetic solutions. Ampoules of local anaesthetic solutions must be packaged and sterilised on the outside to prevent contamination by external glass fragments which often fall inside the ampoule when it is opened. To prevent the possibility of contamination due to withdrawal from small packages, the plastic catheters, taps and syringes required for the 'sterile reservoir system' for continuous epidural analgesia are placed in the composite pack. Cardboard trays prevent distortion of the plastic ware due to high pressure autoclaving.

The hospital pharmacy prepares sterile solutions of local anaesthetic in 60 ml amounts in Honeywell sterile system bottles. This simplifies filling the reservoir syringes. Honeywell bottles have a special sterile lip for pouring which is not contaminated by the fingers when the bottle is opened.

The patient's wishes

Finally, the patient should be an informed and willing subject. In 1970 at the Aberdeen Maternity Hospital 82 patients were asked the following question within the first three days following vaginal delivery: 'Would you have liked to have had your baby without feeling any pain at all during your labour?' The results were as follows:

Multiparae		Primiparae	
Yes	No	Yes	No
17	13	32	20

The wishes of the 40% who expect to feel some pain during labour, and particularly delivery, should be respected. This is important as 31 out of these 33 patients stated that on the whole their labour and delivery was a satisfying experience.

REFERENCES

1. Bonica J J (1967). *Principles and Practice of Obstetric Analgesia and Anesthesia.* Vol. 1 pp. 579, 618, 718 Blackwell, Oxford
2. Crawford J S (1965). *Principles and Practice of Obstetric Anaesthesia.* 2nd Edition p. 208 Blackwell, Oxford

DISCUSSION

Dr Rubin (Charing Cross Hospital, London): May I ask Dr Tunstall why he advocates the paramedian approach exclusively?

Dr Tunstall (in reply): The paramedian approach is just due to an obsession of mine about not damaging the interspinous ligament because I feel that this is a factor in backache.

Complications of Epidural Analgesia

(d) Summing Up

DR C J MASSEY DAWKINS (University College Hospital)

I have been accused of being a prophet of doom because of the number of complications which I have listed, but when one has been doing epidurals for nearly 30 years they do tend to mount up. If one is aware of the existence of complications, then one is far better prepared to deal with them, should they be encountered. Some of them can be extremely bizarre. For example, three patients, under epidural analgesia, breathing spontaneously, oral airways in, under hexobarbitone sedation, their teeth chattered every 5th breath, not every 4th breath, not every 6th breath. My imagination boggles as to the cause. We know many things about epidural block which do not admit of rational explanation. Many of the complications which I have encountered are geriatric ones and are not likely to be met in young women.

Going over the complications briefly, I am surprised that no one has mentioned blood vessel puncture because this is the most common complication of all—2·8%, leading, if unrecognised, to toxic convulsions —0·1%. If you have a needle stuck into the middle of the back and blood is issuing from it, you cannot tell whether you are in the epidural space or not. It has been suggested (believe it or not), that 5 mg of suxamethonium given down the needle would soon solve the question!

With regard to dural puncture one is sometimes appalled at the way registrars in training carelessly enter the theca. I have been informed that at a well-known maternity hospital the junior registrar may expect to puncture the dura four times in his first ten cases, twice in his second ten. This is simply not good enough, it is unfair to the patients. I suggest that it should be mandatory for every junior registrar to spend a month in the neurological department of his hospital learning *how* to do a lumbar puncture so that when he comes to the maternity department he learns how *not* to. One should remember that headache caused by an SWG 16 Tuohy needle is about eight times more frequent than that occurring with an ordinary spinal needle, and that headache may last up to a fortnight.

Table 1

RECORDED CASES		DURAL PUNCTURE
Tactile	30,088	881—2·9%
Visual	13,062	209—1·6%

RECORDED CASES		ACCIDENTAL SPINAL AND/OR MASSIVE EPIDURAL
Tactile	19,537	60—0·3%
Visual	25,774	29—0·1%

The World Dural Puncture Rate, demonstrating the superiority of a visual method of identification of the epidural space.

Table 1 shows the World Dural Puncture Rate, demonstrating clearly that a visual method is more efficient. The discrepancy in the numbers is due to the fact that some authors list complications and others do not; these are only recorded cases where the specific complication has been listed. One has got to trust authors—I remember a well-known American professor getting up at a meeting and saying 'I have done 500 epidurals and I have never punctured the dura'. Discreet enquiries revealed that when he did puncture the dura it became a spinal automatically.

Table 2

RECORDED CASES	DURAL PUNCTURE	ACCIDENTAL SPINAL AND/OR MASSIVE EPIDURAL
5,162	137—2·6%	15—0·3%

Dural Puncture Rate following use of mechanical devices

Table 2 shows that mechanical devices such as the Iklé syringe do not really improve the picture.

Figure 1

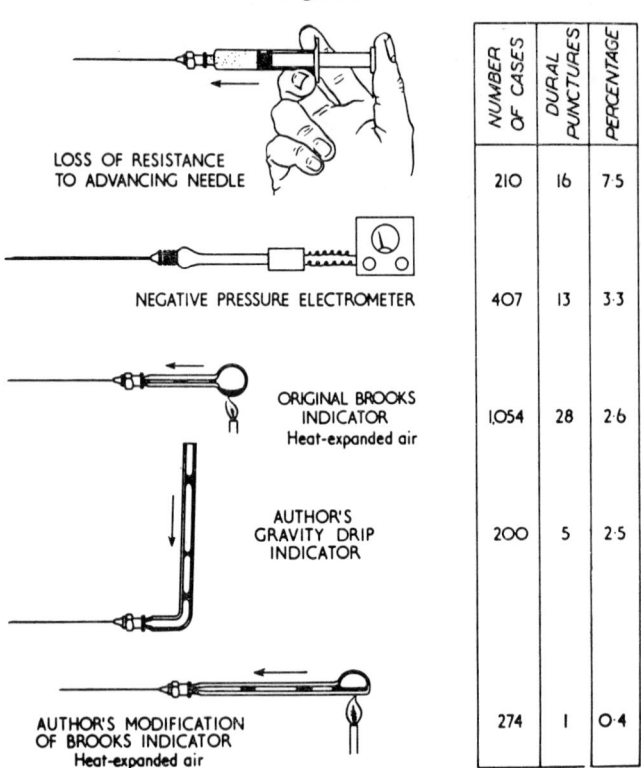

	NUMBER OF CASES	DURAL PUNCTURES	PERCENTAGE
LOSS OF RESISTANCE TO ADVANCING NEEDLE	210	16	7·5
NEGATIVE PRESSURE ELECTROMETER	407	13	3·3
ORIGINAL BROOKS INDICATOR Heat-expanded air	1,054	28	2·6
AUTHOR'S GRAVITY DRIP INDICATOR	200	5	2·5
AUTHOR'S MODIFICATION OF BROOKS INDICATOR Heat-expanded air	274	1	0·4

The author's Dural Puncture Rate in relation to methods used for identification of the epidural space.

Figure 1 shows clearly that the Brooks indicator is much the most efficient and that in my hands I am nineteen times more likely to puncture the dura if I use my thumb than a visual device such as the modified Brooks indicator.

Can I illustrate my point with an analogy. If you had two planes of wood and you were trying to put a metal object between them accurately you wouldn't use a hammer and a nail would you? You would use a screw and a screwdriver. That is why I like to use the Brooks indicator because it does not encumber the needle, you screw it in, it works in 91% of cases and since I started using it with a Tuohy needle I have not yet punctured the dura. If a registrar does his first 20 cases with a visual indicator he will be unconsciously assimilating the feel of the various planes of tissue resistance as his needle goes through. When he is proficient, he can start using his thumb if he prefers it.

Dr Edmonds has mentioned massive epidurals. I have had 13 in 4,300 cases—0·3%. These are very interesting because you have done a perfectly normal epidural. Twenty minutes later the patient slowly stops breathing, the pupils dilate, but the blood pressure does not fall. A piece of cotton wool held over the airway will move in time with the pulse but the patient stays a perfectly normal colour. After a time prudence dictates that you ventilate the patient, it doesn't really seem to be necessary, and after two hours if you have used 2% lignocaine the patient suddenly wakes up, the pupils contract and he is perfectly well. This is quite different from the sequence of events following an accidental spinal. No convincing theory has been advanced as to the cause, I have asked everybody from Bonica and Bromage downwards. They have all had similar cases and no one knows why they occur.

There is no doubt that central nervous system complications do occur. The frequency of permanent neurological damage is about 0·02% and curiously this does not differ from that of a spinal. I believe that, irrespective of where you inject an analgesic solution into the body, trouble may ensue—ask any dentist. He will tell you that he remembers cases of permanent numbness of the lower lip following an inferior dental nerve block. In 785 cases of brachial plexus block that I have managed to find in the literature, there are 27 cases of permanent nerve damage—3·4%, which is very much higher than that of an epidural. So I think that there is no *special* risk if you inject into the epidural space. I have found in the literature 18 cases of permanent damage to the central nervous system. In all these cases adrenaline had been used and I have been unable to find any cases where the specific statement was made that adrenaline had *not* been used. So I would agree with Dr Felicity Reynolds—do we still need adrenaline? I welcome the introduction of bupivacaine without adrenaline.

Finally, remember if you do have neurological trouble it is bound to be blamed on the epidural. My friend Dr Steel was called to Queen Charlotte's Hospital to give an epidural but there was some delay in his arrival. When he got there he found that the patient was being delivered by forceps under nitrous oxide and oxygen analgesia. That patient did not pass urine spontaneously for six weeks afterwards. Dr Edmonds has told you of such a case. I myself have had similar ones. Efforts to get through a bony spine had proved unavailing, the patient was then given a general anaesthetic and next day developed an upper motor neurone lesion. Can anyone doubt that if an epidural had been given in any of these cases the method would have been blamed?

I have had two cases of dural puncture caused by the catheter. It would therefore seem wise to pass the catheter in down the Tuohy needle *before* you do your test dose, because if you give the test dose through the Tuohy needle and all may be well and then you go and puncture the dura with

69

the catheter, disaster will follow. There are many anaesthetists of course who do think that, if you lubricate the epidural space first, the catheter is likely to pass more easily.

Catheters do not always go where they are meant to. Both Sanchez et al[1] and Bridenbaugh et al[2] showed in nearly 300 cases that only 23% of catheters pursue a straight course in the epidural space. 6% pass through an intervertebral foramen, 18% form a single loop and the remaining 53% curl up in the epidural space at the site of insertion.

Figure 2

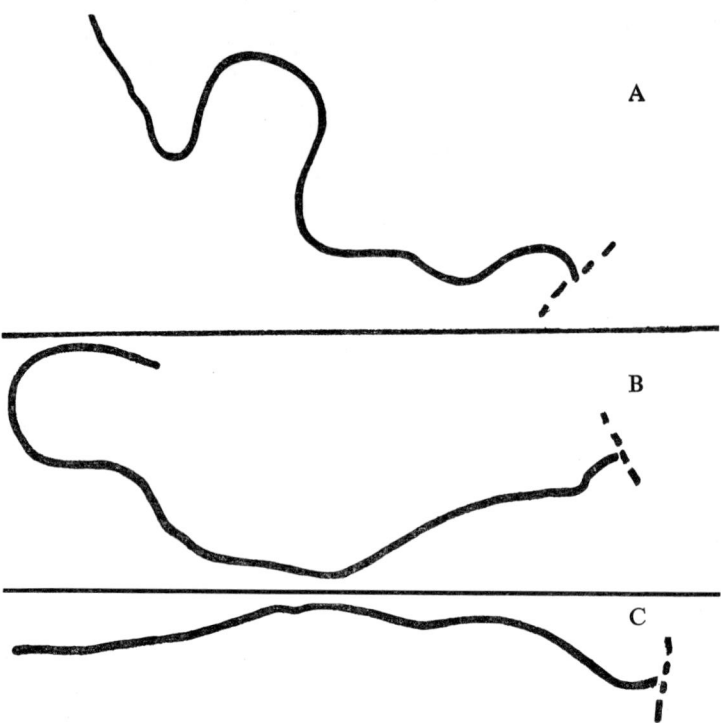

The shape assumed by three vinyl plastic catheters following removal from the patient. Catheters A and B were associated with inadequate analgesia.

Figure 2 shows three catheters of the old vinyl plastic type, which, when you took them out of the body, assumed the shape that they were in in the epidural space. You see the lower one is perfectly all right but inadequate analgesia resulted from injecting down the other two.

Breakage of a catheter is rare, only 0·1%, but there have been three cases of catheters tying themselves into knots. Catheters sometimes come out of the epidural space during labour due to the movement of the patient—just under 2%. Sometimes the patient accidentally pulls them out. Catheters sometimes leak at the junction of the catheter and syringe or at the Millipore filter and I would agree with a previous speaker that a

Tuohy-Borst adaptor is partly the answer to this problem. There really is no perfect solution. If you put the needle inside the catheter you reduce the lumen, if you put the Tuohy-Borst adaptor on you reduce the lumen, if you put a Millipore filter on and seal with a plastic syringe, the syringe all too often breaks. I know that plastic sets have been devised but I continue to use glass syringes because with them not only is there less tendency to break at the nozzle, but also one's sense of tissue resistance is so much more accurate.

Sometimes the catheter gets blocked by a blood clot and I would advise that ½ ml local analgesic solution is injected down the catheter about every 15 minutes.

In my experience of 700 catheters there have been 35 cases when the catheter would not pass; in 23 of those the catheter was passed successfully in the adjacent space so there is an ultimate failure rate of 1·7%.

Now we come to your total failure rate. Gutierrez[3] showed many years ago that the failure rate in his first thousand cases was 6%, his second thousand 3% and his third thousand 0·8%. It is all a matter of practice. There are about five reaons for failure, three caused by the patient and two caused by the anaesthetist. Too bony—can't get the needle through. Too fat—can't find any landmarks, give up; too many blood vessel punctures, give up. Now these are not your fault, they are the patient's fault. Your own fault is, of course, dural puncture and putting in too little local analgesic or putting it in at the wrong place. So to sum up, patient failure rate is 0·9%, human failure rate 0·6%.

It is impossible in the short time at my disposal to cover all the complications that have been encountered. I have tried to list the main ones and to show how they may be avoided.

REFERENCES

1. Sanchez R, Acuna L and Rocha F (1967). *An analysis of the radiological visualization of the catheters placed in the epidural space.* Brit. J. Anaesth. **39**, 485

2. Bridenbaugh L D, Moore D C, Bagdi P and Bridenbaugh P O (1968). Anesthesiology. **29**, 1047

3. Gutierrez A (1932). *Anestesia metamerica peridural.* Buenos Aires.

DISCUSSION

Dr Armstrong (Belfast): I would like to ask Dr Massey Dawkins if he has considered the possibility that bradycardia occurring in babies delivered under epidural analgesia might be due to hypothermia of the baby at birth following maternal heat loss? I have found that post-operative bradycardia in many patients who have undergone relatively long operations almost invariably responds to re-warming in the recovery ward with an electric blanket. Does Dr Massey Dawkins make any attempt to prevent maternal heat loss during continuous epidural analgesia and, if so, how does he do it.

Dr Massey Dawkins (in reply): I must honestly say that I have not thought of this problem. What happens to patients in labour with conventional analgesia? Do they lose heat? I don't know.

Dr Dinnick (Middlesex Hospital): Dr Dawkins has highlighted a theme which has run through the morning's work, namely the question of the need for adrenaline with the local anaesthetic. There is a niggling fear in the back of many of our minds that its use may be related to permanent neurological complications. I would suggest that many people prefer to use 0·25% 'Marcaine' solely because the concentration of adrenaline is less with this solution. Dr Reynolds has already suggested that the need for adding adrenaline is less when bupivacaine is used and I would therefore like to pose the question 'Should we continue to use adrenaline in epidurals?'.

Dr Colback (Newcastle): In considering this matter of changes of body temperature, it more often seems to be one of heat retention rather than heat loss.

Before one is called to give an epidural to a patient in prolonged labour one often finds that considerable quantities of phenothiazine drugs have been given which tend to disorganise the temperature regulating mechanism. The work of labour itself must produce a certain amount of heat and if the ambient temperature is high, these factors must increase body temperature and hence maternal distress.

On the question of the use of adrenaline in epidurals, Pearce[1] reports that the epidural veins are thin walled and contain little or no muscle. Repeated histological examination of epidural veins show them to consist of elastic tissue only. Any increase in the duration of analgesia may be due more to reduced arterial and arteriolar blood flow rather than to a reduced rate of absorption through the venous system. In view of this evidence I do not think that the debate need continue any longer as to whether or not adrenaline should be used with local anaesthetics in the epidural space and I would strongly support those who advocate the use only of plain solutions.

REFERENCE

1. Pearce D J (1957). *The role of posture in laminectomy.* Proc. Roy. Soc. Med. **50,** 109

Indications for Epidural Analgesia with Special Reference to the Management of Pre-Eclampsia

DR DONALD D MOIR (Glasgow)

This paper is based almost entirely on personal experiences with over 2,000 epidural blocks during the past seven years in one large maternity hospital. Indications have been developed jointly with the obstetricians and to some extent by trial and error. We had to modify the extensive experience of transatlantic workers to fit in with a rather different obstetric practice. Seven years ago the British literature on epidural analgesia in obstetrics was confined to a few small series of cases and the service was, to the best of my belief, simply not available, even in many large maternity hospitals.

I must stress that for reasons concerned mainly with staffing we have never pursued a policy of epidural analgesia for every maternity patient. At present we do 400–500 epidurals per annum, so that 12–14% of our patients have this form of pain relief.

The indications fall into three groups:

A. For unusually painful labour.

B. As part of the treatment of pre-eclampsia.

C. Anaesthesia for forceps delivery and Caesarean section.

Indications for 1,800 epidural blocks (Table 1)

Table 1

Continuous Epidural Blocks

Unusually painful labour	1,055 (68%)
Inco-ordinate uterine action	348 (22%)
Severe pre-eclampsia	129 (9%)
Cardiac or respiratory disease	21 (1%)
	1,553

Single-Shot Epidural Blocks

Forceps and Vacuum extraction	214 (92%)
Caesarean section	33 (8%)
	247

A. *Unusually painful labour* is, for this purpose, labour in which pain is not satisfactorily relieved by reasonable doses of narcotic analgesics and inhalational methods. Some idea of the extent of this problem can be obtained from the survey reported by Beazley et al[1] (1967) who found that 40% of women recently delivered were dissatisfied with the pain relief obtained from liberal and early administration of analgesic drugs, including heroin and morphine. These were patients in a teaching hospital and perhaps a more normal group of women would have achieved better relief.

There will be few here today who would deny that epidural analgesia is the most effective method of pain relief in labour. Labour is often unduly prolonged and painful when the occiput is in the posterior position, when uterine action is inco-ordinate or when there is some disproportion. In

73

such labours, the most severe pain is often experienced in the lumbar region and relief of this sometimes agonising backache often seems to require blocking the 2nd, 3rd and 4th sacral nerve roots as well as the 11th and 12th thoracic roots.

Inco-ordinate uterine action is said to exist when labour progresses abnormally slowly due to a dysfunctional type of uterine action. Although the aetiology of this condition is uncertain it is widely held that abnormal and inefficient contractions arise from multiple ectopic foci in the myometrium rather than from the pacemakers at the mouths of the Fallopian tubes. The polarity of the uterus is therefore lost. In the so-called hypertonic variety, contractions are violent and very painful and relaxation between contractions is incomplete. Because the contractions, although powerful, are inco-ordinate, dilatation of the cervix occurs very slowly and descent of the presenting part of the foetus may be delayed.

An association is recognised between inco-ordinate uterine action and cephalo-pelvic disproportion and it is the existence of a definite mechanical problem in about a quarter of these patients which keeps the Caesarean section rate relatively high, particularly in patients living in Glasgow, a city still noted for a high incidence of contracted pelvis. This situation may not apply in the better nourished areas in the South of England.

If inco-ordinate labour persists, then the syndrome of maternal distress develops with the well known features of dehydration, electrolyte deficiencies, ketosis, metabolic acidosis, vomiting, gastro-intestinal distension, tachycardia and pyrexia. There is in vitro evidence that in these conditions uterine action becomes even more inefficient[2].

An external tocodynamometer can be used to demonstrate that in normal labour the uterine contractions occur fairly regularly and are of quite uniform intensity, whereas in inco-ordinate labour, there is a completely erratic pattern of uterine activity with poor relaxation between contractions.

The end result of uterine action in the first stage of labour should be descent of the presenting part and dilatation of the cervix. It is, therefore, easy to assess progress in labour by graphic analysis of the rate of cervical dilatation; a method used extensively by Friedman (1955)[3]. Graphic representation of the rate of cervical dilatation in normal labour produces an S-shaped curve. When labour is inco-ordinate the rate of dilatation is markedly slowed or may even cease altogether. Analysis of 100 successive inco-ordinate labours showed that the rate of cervical dilatation increased at least two-fold in over 70% of patients after the commencement of epidural analgesia and the institution of vigorous intravenous fluid therapy[4].

The traditional management of prolonged and painful labour was 'time and morphia'. Recently Caesarean section has been used much more freely to terminate labour and so relieve the suffering of the mother. In Belfast the Caesarean section rate in inco-ordinate labour has been about 80 per cent for some years, the motives for this high frequency being to terminate the pain. With epidural analgesia labour can continue painlessly, usually with the likelihood of a safe vaginal delivery and Caesarean section can often be avoided in cases of inco-ordinate uterine action not associated with disproportion. This is a particularly worth-while achievement in the young primigravidae who most commonly have inco-ordinate labours.

In over 300 patients with inco-ordinate uterine action managed under, epidural analgesia the Caesarean section rate was 22%. However, in the absence of cephalo-pelvic disproportion the Caesarean section rate fell to 11% and in the smaller group of patients in whom a definite mechanical problem existed, the Caesarean section rate rose to 54%. The perinatal mortality rate in this series of inco-ordinate labours was 1·4%, a low figure for such an abnormal group of patients.

Cardiac or Respiratory Diseases were the primary indication for about 1% of continuous blocks. Severe cardiac disease is not common nowadays in pregnancy. Even so, when pain and anxiety result in tachycardia in the presence of valvular disease, cardiac failure may result from inadequate diastolic filling. I have seen patients in whom epidural analgesia was followed by a slowing of the heart rate and the remission of signs of left ventricular failure. Epidural block is ideal for the forceps delivery which is often indicated in heart disease. In respiratory disease, the avoidance of respiratory depressant drugs is beneficial.

Premature labour, according to several North American authorities, is a specific indication for conduction analgesia (Table 2).

Table 2
The effect of conduction analgesia on perinatal mortality (Ontario Perinatal Mortality Study Committee, 1967)

| | Perinatal Mortality per 1,000 live births | |
	Mature infants	Premature infants
Conduction Analgesia	4·9	140
No Anaesthesia	8·2	440

B. *Treatment of Pre-Eclampsia*

The indication which I would like to discuss in a little more detail is severe pre-eclampsia in labour as we have just completed an assessment of 129 cases in which epidural analgesia was used.

Severe pre-eclampsia is generally agreed to exist when the blood pressure exceeds 160/100 and albuminuria is present, and this was the standard used in this survey.

The cause of pre-eclampsia is unknown and treatment is still directed to the control of various manifestations of the disease.

I submit that the major objectives in treatment are as follows:
(a) to attain a safe blood pressure
(b) to avoid eclampsia
(c) to relieve pain
(d) to avoid deep narcosis
(e) to avoid (further) foetal hypoxia
(f) to maintain urine volume

I also submit, that although some, but not all, of these objectives can be achieved by the older treatments such as that using rectal bromethol, we anaesthetists can surely devise a better regime than full basal narcosis without control of the airway for periods of 24 hours or longer.

Control of Blood Pressure in Pre-eclampsia with Epidural Analgesia
Tables 3 and 4 demonstrate the effect of epidural analgesia in controlling the hypertension in labour of patients with pre-eclampsia.

75

Table 3

Blood pressures in labour of 129 patients with pre-eclampsia *before* epidural block

	B.P. mm Hg	No. of Patients
Systolic Blood Pressure	160–179	85 (66%)
	180–199	30 (23%)
	over 200	14 (11%)
Diastolic Blood Pressure	100–119	85 (66%)
	120–139	38 (29%)
	over 140	6 (5%)

Table 4

Blood pressures in labour of 129 patients with pre-eclampsia *during* Epidural Analgesia

	mm Hg	No. of Patients
Systolic Blood Pressure	Under 140	76 (59%)
	140–159	45 (35%)
	160 plus	8 (6%)
Diastolic Blood Pressure	Under 90	72 (56%)
	90–99	33 (26%)
	100 plus	24 (18%)

Although in general a safe level of blood pressure was maintained during the epidural block, the failure to maintain the diastolic blood pressure below 100 mm.Hg. in 18% of patients is rather disappointing. It should be pointed out, however, that 34% had diastolic pressures in excess of 120 mm.Hg. before the blocks. I believe that hypertension can often constitute a greater risk to the mother's life than eclampsia. Deaths from cerebrovascular accidents still occur.

Eclampsia No patient had a seizure during epidural blockade. Six seizures occurred, in four patients, between 1½ and 8 hours *after* the termination of the block. The lesson is clear; an anticonvulsant drug should have been administered along with the epidural block and should have been continued until all risk of eclampsia had gone. We have had no case of eclampsia since we adopted the anticonvulsant regime of Duffus et al (1969)[5] by giving a continuous infusion of chlormethiazole during the block and often for some hours after delivery. Our practice now implements this concept of balanced therapy by using epidural analgesia to control the blood pressure and relieve pain, in preference to protoveratrine and pethidine.

Perinatal Mortality It is now mainly by perinatal mortality that a therapeutic regime for pre-eclampsia should be judged. Maternal deaths should rarely occur and eclampsia, if it occurs, seldom occurs more than once. Out of the 129 cases in which epidural analgesia was used, 6 (4·6%) infants failed to survive the perinatal period. 4·6% is a low perinatal mortality for severe pre-eclampsia, where dysmaturity and prematurity are common. Perinatal mortality rates of 20% or more were common only 10 years ago. Prematurity and/or placental insufficiency of a severe degree were present in each of the 6 perinatal deaths in this series.

Although epidural analgesia and chlormethiazole infusion do not represent the last word in the management of pre-eclampsia in labour, they constitute a safe, logical and reasonably effective regime. Eclampsia should not occur. Blood pressure will be maintained at a safe level in all but a few patients and the foetus is likely to survive if it is not grossly premature or dysmature.

Some practical points which are perhaps obvious enough, neglect of which have occasionally caused us some trouble are as follows:

(1) Epidural top-ups should be given when the blood pressure rises rather than awaiting the return of pain.

(2) Larger doses may be required—*eg* 10 ml bupivacaine instead of 6–8 ml.

(3) Although control of blood pressure usually prevents eclampsia, it is safer to administer an anticonvulsant drug in addition.

C. *Single-Shot Epidural Blocks for Forceps Delivery or Caesarean Section*
I should like finally to mention briefly the use of single-shot epidural blocks for forceps delivery and Caesarean section. Epidural analgesia is the technique of choice for most forceps deliveries. Occasionally there will be insufficient time to obtain analgesia in acute foetal distress, and perhaps the patient may be quite unsuited to conduction analgesia. The advantages are obvious; the vomiting risk is avoided and drug-induced respiratory depression is eliminated. The condition of the foetus is excellent if hypotension is avoided. The safety of epidural analgesia has far exceeded that of general anaesthesia for operative delivery in several very large American series.

May I remind you of a secondary advantage of epidural analgesia, a substantial and statistically highly significant reduction of blood loss at forceps delivery[6] (Table 5).

Table 5
Blood loss in grams at forceps delivery in relation to different types of anaesthesia [6]

	Average Loss	No. of Patients
Epidural Block	276 ± 57	31
Pudendal Block	412 ± 246	91
General Anaesthesia	518 ± 302	71

I am rather less enthusiastic with epidural analgesia for Caesarean section. Results can be excellent. At other times, nausea and vomiting, associated with traction reflexes or hypotension, can be distressing and difficult to control. Hypotension is a well known hazard of Caesarean section under conduction analgesia. I have used the fluid pre-loading regime advocated by Marx (1969)[7] because it seems logical and is usually effective. One litre of Ringer's lactate solution is given intravenously in the half hour before surgery and a further litre is given during the operation. Very recently we have adopted the practice of performing Caesarean section with a 10 degree left lateral tilt position on the operating table in an attempt to avoid caval compression[8]. All these measures reduce the hazards and the inconveniences of Caesarean section under epidural analgesia, but do not eliminate them.

Contra-Indications to Epidural Analgesia
There are certain generally accepted contra-indications to epidural analgesia. These include infection at the site of puncture, bleeding diseases, anticoagulant therapy, hypovolaemia and gross deformity of the spine. For fear of medico-legal repercussions in the event of a worsening

of the disease it is generally held to be inadvisable to perform epidural analgesia in patients with existing disease of the nervous system.

In addition, there are a number of obstetric conditions in which the technique should be used only after careful consideration of the benefits and the risks:—

(a) *Haemorrhage* The risks of an extensive sympathetic block in the presence of uncorrected hypovolaemia are usually held to contra-indicate epidural analgesia in antepartum haemorrhage and indeed in hypovolaemia from any cause.

(b) *Defibrination* In hypo- or afibrinogenaemia, damage to the epidural veins may cause excessive bleeding and the eventual formation of a large haematoma in the epidural space with the involvement of nerve roots (Hellman, 1965)[9].

(c) *Breech Delivery* Although there are experienced anaesthetists and obstetricians who advocate epidural and spinal analgesia for assisted breech delivery, there are others who avoid these techniques because they fear that perineal anaesthesia and interruption of the involuntary pushing reflex may necessitate breech extraction with its reputedly higher perinatal mortality. A co-operative, intelligent patient can in fact often perform effective voluntary expulsive efforts. Even so, in my experience, breech extraction is sometimes required and perhaps the question at issue is whether breech extraction of a mature, normal infant does indeed carry a much higher perinatal mortality rate than an assisted breech delivery. Certainly, in favour of epidural analgesia is the avoidance of the high risk general anaesthetic which is often requested for delivery of the after-coming head.

(d) *Twin Delivery* In one series of twin deliveries the use of conduction analgesia resulted in a greater mortality rate of the second twin[10]. Others have failed to confirm this observation[11] [12]. It may well be that with any method of anaesthesia the risk to the second twin is greater, and I would regard this point as unsettled. Some of the statements that have been made in the literature are hardly founded on scientific fact or well-controlled series. I am sure that there is a great deal more to this question than the technique of anaesthesia. Prematurity, pre-eclampsia, anaemia and hydramnios are all common in twin pregnancy and obstetricians vary widely in the actual technique of delivery they use. Valid comparisons are therefore difficult and many statements made on either side of this controversy are to be viewed with reservation.

(e) *Previous Caesarean Section* In this situation it is possible that rupture of the uterine scar might be difficult to diagnose. Hypotension and tachycardia might be attributed to the epidural block and pain might be absent.

(f) *Objection by the Patient* Epidural analgesia should never be forced upon an unwilling patient.

REFERENCES

1. Beazley J M, Leaver E P, Morewood J H M and Bircumshaw J (1967). *Relief of pain in labour.* Lancet, **1**, 1033

2. Mark R F (1961). *Dependence of Uterine Muscle Contraction on pH with reference to prolonged labour.* J. Obstet. and Gynaec. Brit. Cwlth. **68,** 584

3. Friedman E A (1955). *Primigravid Labor. A graphico-statistical analysis.* Obstet. and Gynec. **6,** 567

4. Moir D D and Willocks J (1967). *Management of inco-ordinate uterine action under continuous epidural analgesia.* Brit. med. J. **3,** 396

5. Duffus G M, Tunstall M E, Condie R G and McGillivray I (1969). *Chlormethiazole in the prevention of eclampsia and the reduction of perinatal mortality.* J. Obstet. Gynaec. Brit. Cwlth. **76,** 645

6. Moir D D and Wallace G (1967). *Blood Loss at Forceps Delivery.* J. Obst. Gynaec. Brit. Cwlth. **74,** 424

7. Marx G F, Cosmi E V and Wollman S B (1969). *Biochemical status and clinical condition of mother and infant at Caesarean Section.* Curr. Res. Anaesth. **48,** 986

8. Ansari I, Wallace G, Clemetson C A B, Mallikarjuneswara V R and Clemetson C D M (1970). *Tilt Caesarean Section.* J. Obst. Gynaec. Brit. Cwlth. **77,** 713

9. Hellman K (1965). *Epidural Anaesthesia in Obstetrics. A second look at 26,127 cases.* Canad. Anaesth. Soc. J. **12,** 398

10. Little W A and Friedman E A (1958). *Anesthesia for twin delivery.* Anesthesiology, **19,** 515

11. Aaron J B and Halperin J (1955). *Fetal survival in 375 twin deliveries.* Amer. J. Obstet. Gynec. **69,** 794

12. Hingson R A and Hellman L M (1956). *Anesthesia for Obstetrics,* p.251. J.P. Lippincott Company, Philadelphia

DISCUSSION

Dr Ivor Davie (Edinburgh): I would like to say a few words on the management of pre-eclamptic toxaemia. Before we can treat a syndrome it is desirable to know the cause of the syndrome, but unfortunately we do not know the cause of pre-eclampsia. According to Page (1953)[1] eclampsia results when two factors co-exist. The first of these is a sodium sensitisation caused by a high sodium intake in the presence of large quantities of placental steroids and the second is the presence of some vasopressor substance originating from the placenta. Even after many years our knowledge has not progressed much further than that.

The usual treatment of pre-eclamptic toxaemia has been large doses of narcotic and sedative drugs, for example, the so-called lytic cocktail method. These do not always produce satisfactory control of the blood pressure. Basal narcosis with rectal bromethol is commonly used but there is danger of airway obstruction and aspiration of stomach contents. Basically, in pre-eclampsia, treatment should be directed at:

(1) Lowering the blood pressure

(2) Preventing convulsions

(3) Providing analgesia

Ideally, all these things should be done without producing foetal depression.

Scott and Lees[2] have shown that there is usually no increase in cardiac output with pre-eclamptic toxaemia, therefore the increase in blood pressure must be due to an increase in peripheral resistance. In a paper read earlier today, Dr Scott has shown that epidurals seldom affect the cardiac output, the decrease in blood pressure being due to a decrease in the peripheral resistance. It follows therefore, that the reasons for the use of an epidural block in the treatment of pre-eclamptic toxaemia would be that:

(1) it decreases the blood pressure

(2) it relieves pain

(3) it does both these things without producing foetal depression.

Decreasing the blood pressure in severe pre-eclampsia does not invariably prevent eclampsia, but it may be expected to prevent cerebro-vascular accidents, hypertensive encephalopathy and acute left ventricular failure. The use of epidurals does not prevent convulsions and therefore sedation may be necessary.

Dr Moir has already mentioned the use of chlormethiazole and this, I think, is an excellent drug for the purpose of sedation, because it is very easily controllable and there is a very rapid return to consciousness when the administration is stopped. Dr Moir has also shown us that following epidural block there may be a decreased blood loss at delivery which is probably due to the strong retraction of the uterine muscle in the third stage of labour which occurs when the sympathetic nerves are blocked. In pre-eclamptic toxaemia there may be a post-delivery increase in blood pressure and apart from avoiding intravenous ergometrine, I wonder if anyone has had experience in treating this condition. Do they continue with the epidural block or do they use one of the short-acting hypotensives, *eg* phentolamine, trimetaphan or the newer sodium nitroprusside?

Dr Scott (Edinburgh): Dr Moir, have you noticed a post-delivery rise of blood pressure when treating pre-eclampsia with epidural block? We have found this a rather difficult problem as the epidural seems quite unable to control it. A possible solution might be the use of one of the short-acting hypotensive agents.

Dr Moir (in reply): I have also observed post-partum hypertension and have assumed that this was due to a vaso-constrictor effect of ergometrine and an increase in blood volume after placental separation. I have found that an even larger dose of local analgesic is sometimes effective. I would certainly regard the use of bromethol, which I am sure Dr Scott does not advocate, as a retrograde therapeutic measure. It has long been recognised that 25 % of eclamptic seizures occur after delivery.

Dr Fraser Jones (Solihull): I would like to ask for comment on a patient with pre-eclampsia who, despite an effective epidural and chlormethiazole infusion, had severe convulsions while I was actually topping-up the epidural. The baby survived following immediate Caesarean section, but the patient had respiratory inadequacy following operation which necessitated IPPV for a week in the Intensive Care Unit. She recovered completely with excellent renal function and a live baby. Any comment on an obvious mismanagement?

Dr Moir (in reply): My only comment would be that probably the epidural block *had* worn off. I did mention in passing that if you get a good hypotensive effect with bupivacaine, (you do not *always* get an effect), it lasts for only 1½ to 2 hours. The patient is not complaining of pain so if you use pain as your indication for giving top-ups, then you will give them too infrequently. You should give top-ups on the basis of the blood pressure chart.

Dr Colback (Newcastle): I have found in a few cases of pre-eclamptic toxaemia that, following the first top-up dose, a rise of blood pressure no longer occurs before the return of pain and it is therefore no longer the indication for topping-up. Pain may return with the rise of blood pressure or the blood pressure may not rise at all after the waning of analgesia. This suggests that the epidural has eliminated one of the factors, possibly vessel spasm, which has caused hypertension. Has Dr Moir had a similar experience?

Dr Moir (in reply): In my experience what you have described is quite unusual as hypertension tends to get worse as labour progresses. Many patients had very little hypertension before labour but had sudden sharp rises in labour and these rises persisted or were revealed as the epidural block wore off.

Dr Wilson (Leeds): May I ask Dr Moir, with due respect for the potent analgesic properties of bupivacaine, if it would not be reasonable to use lignocaine as the agent of choice in pre-eclamptic toxaemia in view of the apparent greater hypotensive effect that one obtains with it in equi-analgesic dosage? Perhaps Dr Moir has had experience in comparing these two agents in this situation?

With regard to the use of chlormethiazole in conjunction with epidurals, my experience of this has been limited to gynaecological surgery[3]. In this situation, the combination is very successful, with easy control of depth of sedation by adjusting rate of infusion of chlormethiazole. Deep sleep can, however, be obtained with chlormethiazole and even respiratory arrest may result[4]. In the past twelve months two maternal deaths have been brought to my notice due to the inexperienced use of chlormethiazole (in the absence of an epidural, I should emphasise). It is therefore apparent that, although we now have an almost perfect combination of therapeutic agents, even with a safe hypnotic such as chlormethiazole, care in its use must be practised.

Dr Moir (in reply): I did break down these 131 patients into an early group of about 30 who had lignocaine and the other 100 who had bupivacaine. I did not find any clear difference between them in hypotensive effect. Our chlormethiazole dosage is minimal. We do not aim to keep these patients unconscious, we like them to fall into an apparently natural sleep if left alone and to be in a state so that when one speaks to them they will answer without any physical stimulation. This seems to be safe.

Dr Burn (Southampton): Could I ask Dr Moir whether the epidural injection, apart from lowering the maternal blood pressure in pre-eclamptic toxaemia, also has a beneficial effect on the foetus by improving the placental blood supply? I would like to comment too upon the report from Sheffield that 40% of patients were dissatisfied with the degree of pain relief derived from conventional methods of obstetric analgesia (excluding epidural injections). A survey recently conducted at Southampton fully supports such a figure: between 50–60% of patients interviewed found that conventional methods of pain relief were not completely satisfactory. This compares with the group of patients who had been given an epidural injection; of these 100% claimed complete pain relief. I am sure that Sheffield and Southampton are not unique in this respect; they merely reflect the position in the country as a whole.

Finally I should like to ask the obstetricians present if they could add anything to what Dr Moir has said concerning the obstetric contra-indications to epidurals. I have in mind the presence of a classical Caesarean Section scar in the uterus, which might rupture silently; or the presence of a multiple pregnancy when the good uterine retraction following the delivery of the first infant might delay delivery of the twin.

Mr Cooper (Worthing): A contra-indication to using epidural anaesthesia is previous Caesarean Section if the pelvis is small or if you expect any mechanical difficulty. It is not contra-indicated if the previous section was for a non-recurrent case such as placenta praevia. It should not be used if there has been any suggestion of disproportion. I think epidural anaesthesia might add to the difficulties in breech delivery by converting the delivery into a breech extraction. I have no personal experience but I think it might be unwise.

REFERENCES

1. Page E W (1953). *The Hypertensive Disorders of Pregnancy.* Charles C. Thomas, Springfield, Illinois. American Lecture Series

2. Scott D B and Lees M M, Unpublished data

3. Wilson J (1970). Proc. 3rd European Congress of Anaesth. (in press)

4. Wilson J, Stephen G W and Scott D B (1969). *A Study of the Cardiovascular Effects of Chlormethiazole.* Brit. J. Anaesth. **41,** 840

Observations on One Thousand Epidural Blocks Given in Labour

DR J SELWYN CRAWFORD (Birmingham)

If you accept the definition that science is measurement, then this is not a scientific presentation. It is merely a review of certain data which are presented in a numerical fashion, and I make no claim to be able to draw more than the very broadest conclusions from these observations. The data are drawn up from the records of patients who received a lumbar epidural block during labour, subsequent to the introduction of a particular type of record system in our hospital. The first thousand was reached only a couple of weeks ago, and included among these were the records of 55 patients who received an epidural block by infusion of procaine given by a recent colleague of mine, Dr Richmond, who is pursuing that particular problem, and 15 records which could not, in the time available, be matched with the patients' obstetric records. Thus, we have restricted our analysis to the remaining 930 records.

Each patient received bupivacaine, either 0·25% or 0·5% (each with adrenaline), all injections being made via an indwelling catheter. As many of you know, I have a slightly different philosophy from that which has been adopted in most of the other centres in this country. We believe that labour is painful; we believe that epidural analgesia is a remedy for pain, and therefore, unless there are specific contra-indications, epidural block is indicated in each labour. We start off from that premise and look for contra-indications rather than indications. We also believe that a uterine contraction is to some extent painful whether it occurs in premonitory (early), established first-stage or second-stage labour. Therefore, we prefer to cover the entire course of labour with the epidural block, and for that reason we introduce our block as early as possible in labour, or before labour starts.

Table 1

Analysis of the percentage of cases in which the epidural catheter was inserted at various stages of labour

	Time of Insertion of Catheter		
	Before Labour	Premonitory Labour	Established Labour
Primigravid	55	20	25
Multigravid	61	20	19

Table 1 shows that in less than a quarter of the cases an epidural block was instituted when the patient was in established labour. In over half the cases the block was initiated before the onset of labour, and this, of course, is done in conjunction with the induction of labour by artificial rupture of membranes (ARM) and an oxytocin infusion. Our routine is to put in a catheter, induce a perineal block to provide freedom from the pain of the ARM, and then to set up an oxytocin infusion. As soon as the contractions begin, we put in the first dose of bupivacaine through the catheter. I will say—as a provocative aside—that I don't really see the justification for giving a general anaesthetic for an ARM.

The total of patients we are discussing is just over 900, and of these, approximately 600 were primigravidae and just over 300 multigravidae. It is of some interest, I think, to see what was the mode of delivery in these patients (Table 2).

Table 2

Mode of delivery of patients to whom a lumbar epidural block was administered for the relief of pain in labour. In brackets is the percentage of primigravidae and multigravidae delivered in the manner indicated

	Primigravid	Multigravid
Total	591	332
Spontaneous	176 (29·8)	241 (72·6)
Forceps	358 (60·6)	79 (23·8)
Ventouse	16 (2·7)	2 (0·6)
Emergency Caesarean section	41 (6·9)	10 (3·0)

Among the primigravid patients, just under 30% were delivered spontaneously whereas the incidence of forceps delivery was 60%. Among the multigravid patients, almost 73% delivered spontaneously whereas 24% required to be delivered with the aid of forceps. These figures effectively support the theme and suggestions made by our Chairman[1] and many others to the effect that the institution of an epidural block throughout the course of labour need not necessarily lead to mandatory forceps delivery.

Obviously the incidence of forceps delivery and of emergency Caesarean section is dependent upon the patient population, and there is considerable difficulty in attempting to make a comparative analysis with other hospitals—or, indeed, within one's own hospital—among patients who did not receive an epidural block. I would like to make the point that coincidental with the introduction of an epidural service on a large scale in our hospital, there has been a reduction in the incidence of emergency Caesarian section. I do feel that this is one further advantage of the epidurals, that the incidence of emergency section is diminished because of the reduction in maternal and obstetrician's distress.

Further, with reference to the question of the method of delivery, we must take note of the effect of the epidural block upon the bearing-down

Table 3

Percentage incidence of loss of bearing-down sensation among the total series of vaginal deliveries

Mode of Delivery	Primigravid	Multigravid
Spontaneous	45	46
Forceps	74	77

reflex. As shown in Table 3 the bearing-down sensation was abolished in approximately half of the cases in which the delivery was spontaneous, whereas among the patients delivered by forceps, only one quarter retained the bearing-down reflex. Whether or not it is advisable to abolish the bearing-down reflex is a different question: personally, I support the philosophy that an outlet forceps is preferable to a spontaneous delivery from the point of view of both mother and infant. Again with respect to the loss of the bearing-down reflex, our results suggest that the volume of solution injected into the epidural space for the final—pre-delivery—dose does not determine whether or not the bearing-down sensation will be obtunded. However, the response does appear to be concentration-dependent to a quite considerable extent: if 0.5% bupivacaine is used, the loss of bearing-down is far more likely to occur than if 0.25% is used (Table 4).

Table 4

Incidence of loss of bearing-down reflex related to the volume and concentration of the final dose of bupivacaine injected into the epidural space

Final Dose		Percentage Loss of Bearing-Down Reflex
Vol. (ml)	Concentration (Per Cent)	
< 6	0·25	58
	0·50	71
6	0·25	40
	0·50	72
8	0·25	58
	0·50	70
> 8	0·25	56
	0·50	81

Now we come to the crux of the matter—the extent of patient approval, (Table 5). We visit each patient on the day after her delivery and record

Table 5

Patient's assessment (elicited on the first post-natal day) of the efficiency of the epidural block during labour and at delivery. The figures refer to the percentage in each category

	Primigravid	Multigravid	Total
Fully Satisfied	84	75	81
Helped	10	16	12
No Benefit	6	7	6
Satisfaction + Deprivation	1 (6 Patients)	1 (3 Patients)	1

the extent of her approval, using one of four categories: we ask if she was fully satisfied, whether she feels she was helped, whether the epidural was of no benefit, and a final question to which I will refer later. Obviously this is a very crude type of analysis, but I am not prepared to go into any greater detail within the context of clinical observation and for the purpose of carrying out a clinical service. I ask you to take my word for it that

85

when a patient is recorded as having been fully satisfied, she has not only said that she has been satisfied, but she has usually appended remarks such as 'It was a marvellous thing and are you sure I can come back here for the next one and have the same again?' This sort of remark is undoubtedly very frequently heard during the ward rounds, and I have no hesitation in saying 'fully satisfied' does indeed mean that there has been virtually total pain relief.

I would like to draw attention to the small group of patients who comprise the category 'Satisfaction plus deprivation'. These patients command a considerable amount of respect. They have declared themselves as having been freed from pain during labour and delivery, but said that they would not have an epidural again because of the feeling of having failed in their duty or having failed to participate in labour and delivery, or that there was 'something missing'. Whatever attitude one adopts privately to that sort of emotional response, one most certainly has to respect it, and it occurs in approximately 1 % of our patients. That, of course, is 1 % of the patients who have said that they would have an epidural block: there is quite a number of patients who refuse to have an epidural block because of this particular emotional attitude towards the pain of labour.

We have an internal check on the efficiency of the block inasmuch as we make note of the effect of a single dose of the agent when we come to do a top-up. Under these circumstances, the patient is still in labour and if she has had pain during the previous one or two hours she is certainly going to tell you about it. There is no question of loss of recall of painful episodes, we are making note of on-the-spot assessment by the patient. Here (Table 6) is the incidence of top-up doses, excluding the final dose.

Table 6

Patient's assessment of the efficiency of each injection of bupivacaine (excluding the final one before delivery) obtained at the time of injection of the succeeding top-up

Dose (ml)	Concentration (Per Cent)	No. of Doses	Pain Abolished (Per Cent)	No Relief (Per Cent)
< 6	0·25	107	57	7
	0·50	53	51	8
6	0·25	125	71	2
	0·50	64	53	17
8	0·25	1,868	82	3
	0·50	307	86	1
> 8	0·25	467	82	2
	0·50	52	73	10

As you see, the effectiveness of pain-relief appears to be volume-related and not concentration-related, and we have settled upon the choice of 8 ml of 0·25% bupivacaine for the routine top-up dose. When 8 ml or more is injected, on more than 80% of occasions complete relief from pain is provided. This correlates quite well with the assessment made with reference to the retrospective analyses on the day after delivery. The opinion is further strengthened by an analysis of the efficiency of the final dose in respect to relieving pain at the end of labour and during delivery

Table 7

Patient's assessment of efficiency of final dose of bupivacaine to be injected before delivery—obtained shortly after delivery

	Efficiency During Delivery				
	Final Dose				
Vol. (ml)	Concentration (Per Cent)	No.	Mean Time Pre-Delivery (Min.)	Discomfort (Per Cent)	Pain (Per Cent)
< 6	0·25	30	65	17	0
	0·50	26	65	23	12
6	0·25	37	46	11	11
	0·50	24	57	17	8
8	0·25	336	74	11	4
	0·50	120	73	8	6
> 8	0·25	116	72	8	4
	0·50	23	75	4	0

(Table 7), from which we again conclude that the volume of drug injected is more important than is the choice of concentration in determining the success of the block. In reference to the failure to relieve pain, I have to report that in approximately 6% of patients, additional analgesia had to be given to provide relief from pain during first-stage labour, and that 7% of patients required additional analgesia during the second-stage and at delivery.

We have analysed the duration of effectiveness of the topping-up doses and have come to the same conclusion as others, that irrespective of the concentration of the bupivacaine used or of the volume, the mean duration of activity is approximately 120 minutes. In the post-delivery period, however, the sensory loss is considerably longer, lasting for approximately four hours. There has been no effect upon the duration of the first stage of labour irrespective of whether the patients are primigravid or multigravid, or whether the epidural was started before the onset of labour or when labour was on the point of becoming established.

Finally, I would like to talk about the complications that we have met. We have a total of 71 dural taps out of this 1,000-odd cases, an incidence of approximately 7%. I accept that this is high when compared with that expected in an efficiently-run service staffed by people who are already trained to do epidurals. Because we are the only hospital in the United Birmingham Hospitals doing epidurals, I have to teach on the worst patients of all—the pregnant patients. We have to accept this incidence, we hope that this will change later. Certainly the incidence of dural taps is well correlated with inexperience; of the patients given an epidural by a doctor who had done fewer than 10, 13% were given a dural tap. Amongst those who were given an epidural block by somebody who had done between 10 and 50 epidurals, 6% got a dural tap. Where the experience of the anaesthetist exceeded the 60 mark, 2% of the patients got a dural tap. We have recorded that of the 71 dural taps, 9 were initiated with the catheter. Now that is pure impression of the anaesthetist because he or she felt that the catheter, and not the needle, went through the theca. Cerebro-spinal fluid was not observed to flow back through the needle in these cases, but was seen to flow back through the catheter either at the time that the catheter was threaded beyond the tip of the needle or within a period up to several minutes after placement of the catheter. You can argue about that as long as you like, but we merely have it down on the records as an impression of people who were at the site of action.

Of the 71 patients who received a dural tap, 16 had no headache, which I find a rather surprising figure. I had assumed that nearly everybody would get a headache but 16 of the patients had no headache in the six days that we followed them up subsequent to delivery. 37 of the 71 had headache on the first and successive days, 9 more did not start until the second day. Amongst the patients who had no dural tap but still had an epidural, the incidence of headaches was again remarkably high. We are looking into this, most patients blame it on the central heating in the hospital.

Hypotension was discussed at length this morning and all I would like to say is that amongst our thousand patients I have records of only four patients who definitely had hypotension referable to autonomic blockade. Among the other complications, if they can be so called, is backache, which occurs so frequently in obstetric patients that I do not really feel that it has much to do with the epidural; 50% of patients had a backache during the first six days after delivery. Another is bladder disturbance, which we characterise most frequently as being a loss of bladder sensation. Our patients say that they empty their bladder as it were by the clock. The incidence of this is definitely related to the degree of trauma of delivery. It has been found to occur in 25% of forceps deliveries and in 11% of spontaneous deliveries, being noted on the first or second or on both the first and second post-delivery days.

REFERENCE

1. Doughty A (1969). *Selective Epidural Analgesia and the Forceps Rate.* Brit. J. Anaesth. **41,** 1058

DISCUSSION

The Chairman: I am interested that you had a fair number of patients that were not satisfied with the pain relief and I am wondering whether the anaesthetist concerned pursued the matter hard enough to try to get the epidural to work. I am thinking particularly of a certain number of patients in whom the block is initially unilateral and if you turn them on to the unaffected side and give supplementary doses of local anaesthetic through the catheter most of them get relief. Some of them do not, and I find in these cases satisfactory analgesia is only obtained by removing the cannula and making a fresh epidural puncture in another lumbar inter-space. I do not know whether you would call that a failure of block, although ultimately you satisfy the patient because you are determined to do so. I do not think that anyone ought to set out to give epidural analgesia unless he is determined to be satisfied with nothing less than complete pain relief for the patient.

The second point is that, with your experience of dural taps, no doubt caused by your junior colleagues, I would like to know how you manage the patients afterwards. Is there anything more you can do than to keep them lying flat perhaps for a week or ten days until they can sit up without a return of headache?

The third point I would like to ask is this. Am I right in believing that you use straight needles in preference to Tuohy needles and therefore your catheters are pointing straight at the dura instead of being inclined at an angle to it? Might not this be related to the large number of dural taps? In addition do you train your juniors not to pass the catheter during a contraction while the dura is tense and therefore more liable to puncture?

Dr Crawford (in reply): We do avoid advancing the epidural needle during a contraction and, in any case, only 25% of our patients were in labour when the catheter or needle were introduced. We do use a straight, short-bevelled needle.

With respect to the patients who have not been fully satisfied; the figures reflect the fact that we have been trying to be honest. If the effectiveness of one or two top-ups in the series of six or eight has been less than satisfactory then that patient is designated as having been merely 'helped' during labour. She has not been fully satisfied because the pain relief has not extended throughout the whole of labour. Most certainly we do get an incidence of unilateral block and of unblocked segments. We have had three or four patients with absolutely classic unilateral blocks which we have not been able to satisfy. We have had more which we have been able to overcome by appropriate positioning. We have had an incidence of something that is not referred to in the literature; a patch of pain in one or other groin that is apparently related to the ilio-hypogastric distribution, and I cannot explain that because the ilio-hypogastric nerve does not form until it gets outside the epidural space.

As to the management of patients who have had an inadvertent dural tap; we started off in the classical manner, we kept the patients lying down, we encouraged them to drink as much as possible. It was certainly very impressive to me meeting this thing on a large scale for the first time, to see how well the classic description was fulfilled. I found that there was a small number of nine-day headaches but for the majority you could with increasing assurance say to a patient: 'This will stop tomorrow or the day after tomorrow' whenever the sixth day arises. Now we have instituted further methods. As soon as dural tap is obtained, we give the patient a litre of Hartmann's solution straight away after the epidural catheter has been successfully inserted. Only eleven of those taps were actually abandoned cases; in the remaining 60 we went on to do an epidural. That is the most important thing: seeing that the patient is given a pain-free labour and does not bear down at all and has an outlet forceps. We give them a litre of Hartmann's solution immediately after the epidural is going, give them another litre the next day. We make sure that the patients have a very soft and easy bowel action on the third day because if they strain at stool on the third day I feel sure that they can pop open a repairing hole in the dura and start their headache then. We are now leaving the catheter in and seeing what is the effect of giving the saline into the epidural space during the post-natal period.

As an aside may I mention that at least up to the 10th to 14th dose we have found no evidence of tachyphylaxis with regard to bupivacaine.

Mr Frampton (Warwick): I am a little worried by the number of patients who are being given the epidural injection before the onset of labour. I know that it is unusual for someone to fail to induce labour surgically but it does happen once in a while. Indeed having ruptured the membranes there is a small group of women who will not go into labour regardless of an oxytocin infusion. I feel therefore that you have subjected someone to a technique which may well be harmless but nevertheless unnecessary unless you are going to proceed to do a Caesarean section under epidural block. I wonder if perhaps you had thought of that.

May I ask a second question? Do you feel that up and down the country junior or middle grade obstetric personnel could be trained to use this technique, and indeed should be, in view of the comparative shortage of anaesthetists in the district hospitals as compared with the teaching centres?

Dr Crawford (in reply): You are quite right. There is a small number of patients in whom the induction of labour fails so you are left with a patient with an epidural catheter in her back. You have given her the relief of pain for the amniotomy but you might have to abandon the method. It is very likely that you are going to make another attempt to initiate labour the next day. You are not going to leave a patient with ruptured membranes for more than 24 to 36 hours even is she is not in labour. Now the epidural catheter can be left in for six or seven days without causing any apprehension to the anaesthetist or discomfort to the patient. It can be left in until the next day. I do not think that there is a formidable objection to this particular method of conducting the service. Furthermore, if Caesarean section is undertaken because of failure to induce labour, the route into the epidural space can be used to provide anaesthesia for the operation although we do not ourselves use this technique; the indwelling catheter can also be used to provide post-operative analgesia.

With regard to your second question, that raises a matter which is of concern to the Obstetric Anaesthetists' Association in its business capacity. We hope to discuss matters of this order later, but I would draw your attention to the fact that there are plenty of consultant anaesthetists now in this country, not immediately attached to or in the vicinity of a teaching hospital, who are running their own epidural services; this is not a high-falutin' service, this is a service which anaesthetists should make available in all hospitals with maternity departments delivering more than 2,000 mothers a year. I would not object personally to the obstetricians doing it, in fact I teach obstetric registrars who want to learn, but the facilities for observation and supervision by the anaesthetic service should be immediately available.

The Choice Between the Lumbar and Caudal Route

Dr A P Rubin (Charing Cross Hospital)

Introduction

Continuous caudal analgesia was introduced into obstetrics by Hingson and Edwards in 1942[1], although the single dose method had been used since 1909[2]. It is widely practised in some countries to provide analgesia for labour and delivery, and this paper describes some of my experiences with the technique during a year spent in the United States.

A method of caudal analgesia will be outlined. The success rate and the effects on maternal blood pressure and on labour will be described. Finally the caudal and lumbar routes will be compared and contrasted.

Method

To institute caudal analgesia, the patient is usually placed in the lateral Sims position. If the landmarks are not readily apparent, they may be more easily identified if the knee-chest, or the prone position with a bolster under the pelvis is used. However, these positions are uncomfortable and less acceptable to the parturient.

May I review briefly the landmarks for caudal block. The structures that should be identified are the coccyx, sacral cornua, and the posterior superior iliac spines (Figure 1). In most patients the sacral hiatus lies 2 to

Figure 1

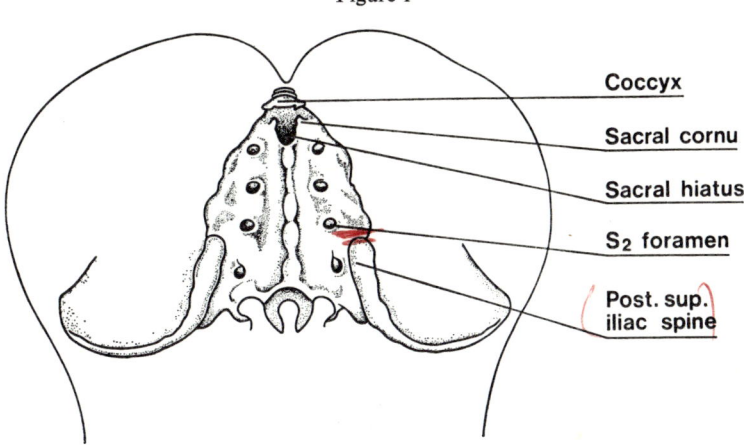

Coccyx

Sacral cornu

Sacral hiatus

S₂ foramen

Post. sup. iliac spine

The Anatomy of Caudal Injection

2½ inches (5–6 cm) from the tip of the coccyx, and a finger tip passed along the coccyx from its distal end will usually drop into the hiatus. Furthermore, the hiatus may be assumed to lie at the apex of an equilateral triangle whose base is a line joining the posterior superior iliac spines.

The second sacral foramina are situated ½ inch (1 cm) medial and ½ inch (1 cm) inferior or caudal to the posterior superior iliac spines (Figure 1). An estimate of their position gives a useful guide to the level to which the dural sac may descend, and the caudal needle should not be inserted beyond this point.

The caudal area should be thoroughly cleaned, prepared with an antiseptic solution, and covered with sterile towels. It is essential to prevent contamination of the puncture site by faeces, liquor or urine. The block is performed using full aseptic technique.

Once the hiatus has been located, it is important to keep pressure with the thumb on the upper margin of the hiatus to prevent movement of the skin over the underlying structures. This is particularly essential with the more obese patient in the lateral position, as otherwise the midline skin crease will tend to sag, and it is very easy to insert the needle laterally. Furthermore, once the skin and subcutaneous tissues have been infiltrated, the landmarks tend to become obscured.

After infiltration a 25 swg needle is used to seek the characteristic drop through the sacrococcygeal membrane on to the periosteum of the anterior sacral bone, and once this has been found an 18 swg thin-walled needle is inserted.

When the sacrococcygeal membrane has been pierced, the hub of the needle is depressed towards the natal cleft, and the needle advanced in the midline under the posterior surface of the sacral canal. By keeping the needle posteriorly, one hopes to avoid the large thin-walled veins which are most numerous anteriorly, and also the rough transverse ridges, often present on the anterior wall of the canal, which can impede the advancement of the needle. The direction in which the needle should be advanced may be estimated by feeling for the lumbar spines, as the angle of inclination of the sacral canal may be about 15 or 20 degrees to the horizontal.

Once the needle is inserted, careful aspiration for blood or cerebrospinal fluid is made. Should blood be obtained, the needle is repositioned until no more blood can be aspirated. If cerebrospinal fluid is obtained, it is safest to abandon the procedure. No fluid having been aspirated, a test injection of air or saline is made. A mass will be felt if the needle has been placed subcutaneously. If the point of the needle is under the periosteum of the sacrum, there will be great resistance to the injection and the patient usually experiences considerable pain. With correct placement of the needle, there will be complete lack of resistance to the injection.

A catheter with wire stylet is passed through the needle, aiming to place the catheter tip at the level of the fifth lumbar vertebra. If the catheter tip is left in the sacral canal, much of the local analgesic agent injected passes out through the large anterior sacral foramina. These are not covered with muscle or ligament, and some of the local analgesic passes out through them before it can effect blockade within the sacral canal. However, if the local analgesic can be injected at the fifth lumbar level, there is less leakage and the dose required to produce analgesia to the tenth thoracic segment can be kept to a minimum.

The stylet and the caudal needle are withdrawn, and the catheter connected to a Tuohy-Borst adaptor (Figure 2). This adaptor, which has a sterile cap, conveniently solves the problem of keeping the catheter tip sterile, and facilitates top-up injections. A bacterial filter may be inserted.

Figure 2

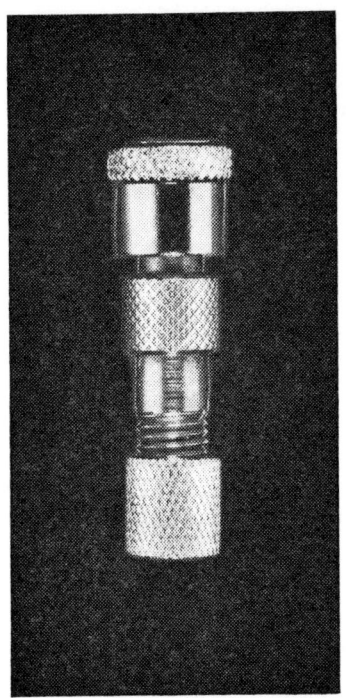 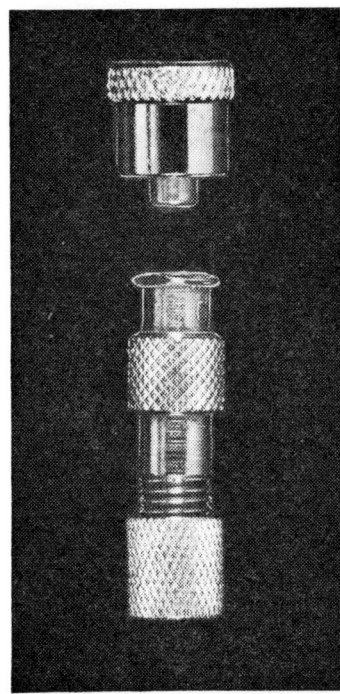

The Tuohy-Borst Adaptor (a) with cap on (b) with cap off showing the Luer-Lock hub.

After aspiration is repeated, and no blood or cerebrospinal fluid obtained, a 3 ml test dose of 1% lignocaine or 1% mepivacaine with 1 in 200,000 adrenaline is made, to ensure that the catheter is not in the subarachnoid space or in a blood vessel. After five minutes, this is followed by the therapeutic dose of the same solution. An average dose of 18 ml was used, being varied if the patient was much above or below average height. Bupivacaine had not been released by the Food and Drugs Administration in 1969, and so I was not in a position to use it. However, I consider it to be the agent of choice for continuous caudal analgesia for the relief of pain in labour, because of its longer duration of action and relatively poor motor blockade.

Analgesia would usually begin within ten minutes, but in about 10% of patients the onset would be delayed for twenty minutes or even half an hour. The onset of caudal analgesia is often said to be slower than with the lumbar approach as the injection site is farther from the lower thoracic segments[3].

Success Rate

The success rate of caudal block is usually thought to be somewhat low due to the frequent anomalies of the sacral canal and hiatus and the difficulty of identifying the landmarks in the more obese subject. A summary of the results of my first 100 continuous caudals performed in the United States over a six week period are shown in Table 1. A block

Table 1

Success Rate of Continuous Caudal Block with increasing experience

Numbers	Successful	Percentage
1–20	14	70%
21–40	17	85%
41–60	18	90%
61–80	19	95%
81–100	19	95%

was called successful if there was demonstrable sensory loss to pin prick, although about 10% of these patients still experienced some discomfort in the back, abdomen or thighs, or an unpleasant dragging sensation if the forceps were used. It will be seen that once the technique has been mastered, a success rate of about 95% can be expected, and similar success rates have been achieved by other workers[4][5]. However I am sure that with equal experience in the two techniques, the success rate of lumbar epidurals is even higher, and this has been reported in many series[3][6].

Effect on Maternal Blood Pressure

The effects of caudal block on maternal blood pressure seem to be very similar to those of the lumbar route, and I will not dwell for long on this aspect, as it has been discussed at some length by previous contributors to this symposium. The fall in blood pressure with these techniques seems to be mainly related to the height of the block, and hence the extent of sympathetic blockade produced. Also, acute dilatation of the vasculature of the lower limbs caused by the sympathetic blockade, accentuates the effect of inferior vena caval obstruction by the gravid uterus and may aggravate the hypotension.

About 40% of the patients show less than a 10 mm.Hg fall in systolic pressure, while about 70% show less than a 20 mm.Hg fall (see Table 2). Only a very few show a drop greater than 30 mm.Hg and most of these are hypertensive or toxaemic subjects.

Table 2

Fall in Blood Pressure with Caudal Block

Fall (mm.Hg)	Percentage
10	40%
10–20	30%
20–30	20%
30	10%

The hypotension is usually completely corrected by placing the patient in the lateral position or by left uterine displacement. If a vasopressor is required, ephedrine appears to be the most suitable, as it produces a rise in maternal blood pressure and an improvement in foetal condition.[7]

Effects on Labour

In the United States the block is traditionally started when the patient is in the active phase of labour, and the cervix five to six centimetres dilated in the primigravida or four to five centimetres dilated in the multigravida. It is however often started earlier if there is inco-ordinate uterine action or if the patient is complaining of considerable pain.

Some authorities, including a previous contributor to this symposium,[8][9] advocate placement of the epidural catheter early in labour, or even at the time of an induction of labour, as it is easier to perform the block when the patient is not distresssed or restless; it can then be used to provide analgesia for the induction or it can be injected immediately it is required. I think that it is unwise to insert the catheter too early as circumstances may change, and it may not be indicated later in labour. One such patient had a caudal catheter inserted which was not used over the course of her labour. When the time came to remove it, the catheter was found to be fractured below skin level, and on surgical exploration, the whole severed fragment was lying within the sacral canal. I feel that it is better to await the onset of the active phase of labour before commencing the block, and I suggest that the patient would tolerate the procedure much better when urgently awaiting pain relief.

The effects on the first stage of labour seem to be minimal and very similar to those of lumbar epidurals[10][11]. However, caudal block does reverse the desirable sequence of blockade, producing perineal analgesia before it is required, and possibly the early abolition of reflexes from the cervix which have been thought to be a factor in the normal progress of labour.

The second stage is usually prolonged due to the total lack of any desire to bear down. There may be a decrease in the complete rotation of the foetal head resulting in an increase in persistent occipito-posterior or transverse positions[12][13]. The incidence of forceps delivery is usually high, although in the U.S.A. this is often from choice. Spontaneous delivery can be achieved with caudal analgesia especially if weak concentrations of local analgesic are used, but it entails considerable determination and co-operation on the part of the mother and her attendants.

Advantages and Disadvantages

The advantages and disadvantages of caudal analgesia when compared with the lumbar route are presented in Table 3.

Table 3
Continuous Caudal Analgesia—A Comparison with Lumbar Epidural

Advantages	Disadvantages
1. More comfortable position	1. Increased failure rate
2. Less painful and more rapidly instituted	2. Larger doses of local analgesic
3. Very low incidence of dural puncture, hence headache or total spinal very rare	3. Slower onset of analgesia
4. Perineal analgesia always present	4. Inability selectively to block first stage pain pathways
5. Patient acceptance	5. Increased forceps delivery rate
	6. Increased liability to infection
	7. Risk of puncturing foetal head
	8. Coccydynia

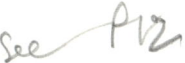 See P12

95

The first advantage of caudal analgesia is that it may be performed with the patient in a more comfortable position. As no flexion of the spine is required, and the procedure is rather less painful and more rapidly instituted, it is the easier route if the patient is restless or not fully co-operative.

Dural puncture is very rare, so that total spinal is less likely to occur. This is a factor of the greatest importance in obstetric centres where those other than anaesthetists wish to employ regional block techniques. Similarly, post-dural puncture headache is equally unlikely.

Perineal analgesia is always obtained, whereas this may be deficient with the lumbar route unless the patient is sat up for some time to allow the local analgesic to gravitate to the second, third and fourth sacral segments.

Finally, a few patients will accept caudal analgesia while refusing the lumbar approach due to the fear of a needle inserted into the lumbar spine and its consequences.

The disadvantages of the caudal approach include firstly the increased failure rate which has already been discussed, and the fact that the patient receives a much larger total dose of local analgesic drug over the course of labour. This could lead to an increased blood level of local analgesic agent and might result in maternal or foetal toxicity.

Following administration of lignocaine in the epidural space, umbilical vein levels of the drug above $3\mu g/ml$ may be associated with depressed babies at birth as judged by the Apgar score[14].

The possible slower onset of analgesia, the inability selectively to block first stage pain pathways which pass to the eleventh and twelfth thoracic segments, and the increased forceps rate have all been discussed.

An increased liability to infection is always suggested as the puncture site lies so close to the perineum. Also the rectum can be entered by a misplaced needle with resulting infection if the contaminated needle is then placed in the sacral canal.

Another disadvantage of caudal analgesia is the risk of accidentally puncturing the foetal skull and even injecting a mass of local analgesic into the foetal brain[15]. In view of this very rare but catastrophic complication, which is invariably due to inserting the caudal needle lateral to the sacrum or coccyx, some authorities do not recommend caudal block in late labour when the foetal head is low in the pelvis[3].

Finally, coccydynia is an occasional post-partum complaint, and if a caudal block has been administered, it will usually be related to it in the patient's mind.

Conclusions

Caudal block is a convenient and successful method of providing analgesia for labour and for assisted vaginal deliveries. In the hands of those experienced in its use, it is extremely safe, the results are excellent, and it has relatively few complications.

The lumbar route is usually preferred for prolonged pain relief in the first stage of labour because it is anatomically more logical, and requires smaller doses of local analgesic agent. However the caudal route has some advantages, which have been outlined, and is indicated in certain patients.

The continuous technique is advocated because it provides much greater flexibility of the duration, extent, and intensity of the block, and allows the smallest effective amount of local analgesic to be used.

Caudal block has a definite place in the repertoire of the obstetric anaesthetist. It can be wisely adopted in selected patients for the relief of pain in labour, and offers a safe alternative to subarachnoid block or general anaesthesia for some obstetric procedures.

REFERENCES

1. Hingson R A and Edwards W B (1942). *Continuous Caudal Anesthesia During Labor and Delivery*. Curr. Res. Anesth. Analg. **21**, 301

2. Stoeckel D (1909). *Sakrale Anästhesia*. Zentralbl. Gynäk, **33**, 3

3. Bonica J J (1970). *In Obstetrical Anesthesia. Current Concepts and Practice*. Editor Sol. M Shnider, Williams and Wilkins, Baltimore 1970, p.75

4. Bush R C (1959). *Caudal Analgesia for Vaginal Delivery. II. Analysis of Complications*. Anesthesiology, **20**, 186

5. Bonica J J (1967). *Principles and Practice of Obstetric Analgesia and Anesthesia*. Vol. 1, p. 574, F A Davis Company, Philadelphia

6. Hehre F W and Sayig J M (1960). *Continuous Peridural Anesthesia in Obstetrics*. Amer. J. Obstet. Gynec. **80**, 1173

7. Shnider S M, de Lorimier A A, Hill J W, Chapler F K and Morishima H O (1968). *Vasopressors in Obstetrics*. Amer. J. Obstet. Gynec. **102**, 911

8. Nohill W K and Howland R S (1958). *Pitocin-Caudal Anesthesia Method of Artificial Induction of Labor*. New York J. Med. **58**, 198

9. Crawford J S In this Symposium p. 83

10. Vasicka A and Kretchmer H (1961). *Effect of Conduction and Inhalation Anesthesia on Uterine Contractions*. Amer. J. Obstet. Gynec. **82**, 600

11. Caldeyro-Barcia R and Poseiro J J (1960). *Physiology of the Uterine Contraction*. Clin. Obstet. Gynec. **3**, 386,

12. Ritmiller L F and Rippman E T (1957). *Caudal Analgesia in Obstetrics: Report of Thirteen Years Experience*. Obstet. Gynec. **9**, 25

13. Friedman A, Schantz S and Pace H R (1960). *Continuous Caudal Analgesia and Anesthesia in Obstetrics. A Critical Evaluation of 510 cases*. Amer. J. Obstet. Gynec. **80**, 1181

14. Shnider S M and Way E L (1968). *Plasma Levels of Lidocaine (Xylocaine) in Mother and Newborn following Obstetrical Conduction Anesthesia: Clinical Applications*. Anesthesiology, **29**, 951

15. Finster M, Poppers P J, Sinclair J C, Morishima H O and Daniel S S (1965). *Accidental Intoxication of the Fetus with Local Anesthetic Drug during Caudal Anesthesia*. Amer. J. Obstet. Gynec. **92**, 922

DISCUSSION

The Chairman: Thank you, Dr Rubin, for putting the case for and against the caudal route in such a balanced and unprejudiced fashion. It has always seemed odd to me that, in this country, most of the practitioners of caudal analgesia seem to be obstetricians while anaesthetists tend to use the lumbar route. All descriptions of caudals prescribe the use of a test dose and yet there is said to be lower liability to dural puncture, while few appear to advocate a test dose with lumbar epidurals and yet presumably the incidence of dural puncture is greater than with caudals.

I was also interested in your observation that you can obtain loss of cutaneous sensation up to the lower dorsal dermatomes and yet have imperfect relief of labour pain. With lumbar epidurals one often obtains perfect relief of labour pain with imperfect loss of cutaneous sensation. Can you account for this?

Dr Rubin (in reply): I think that the use of a test dose merely reflects a difference in transatlantic practice. In most centres in the United States test doses are used with both the lumbar and caudal techniques. In this country, although some workers do recommend test doses, it would seem that most do not with either route.

I cannot say that it has been my experience that one obtains perfect relief of labour pain with imperfect loss of cutaneous sensation. I think that even with the lumbar route I have found patients in whom analgesia to pinprick was present to the tenth thoracic segment, and who still complain of some pain or discomfort, very commonly in the lower abdomen or groins.

The Chairman: My main point was to elicit your views as to why the lumbar route is considered so difficult and the caudal route so easy, so easy in fact that even obstetricians can do caudals. Yet anaesthetists are somewhat loath to start on the caudal route which I think is probably more difficult. After all you only have one sacral hiatus to penetrate and if you cannot find that one hole you have to abandon your attempt to do a caudal. In the lumbar region you have a choice. If you cannot penetrate one lumbar interspace you can attempt the puncture in another.

Dr Rubin (in reply): I do not think that it is a question of being easy or difficult, rather one of tradition. There are many centres, as in Oxford in this country, where the obstetricians have set the pace in the regular use of caudal block in labour. I think that the preference of the obstetricians for this route is based on the belief that it is the safer route, as there is less risk of dural puncture and resulting total spinal blockade.

Dr Nicholas (Sheffield): I do not want to be thought discourteous but I think every series of caudal blocks that I have come across are always in selected patients. In other words, the sacral hiatus has to be identifiable before you should attempt the block. I now only do caudals when I am very sure of success because I know I can penetrate the epidural space with certainty in the lumbar region. I work with two obstetricians who were trained in Oxford, where caudals have been done for fifteen years and the method has worked very well. These colleagues are now giving up caudals and are using the lumbar route, not only because they find it so much easier, but also because of the higher success rate, the lower dose of local analgesic used and because the procedure is less painful to the patient. The only inadvertent dural tap done by the obstetricians in our hospital was in attempting a caudal block and they have never yet produced a dural tap by the lumbar route. We have had only two in nearly four years. I think that providing there is adequate cover for those who are learning it is unlikely to happen and our obstetricians are very much happier doing lumbar epidurals and they do them very well.

I cannot agree with Dr Rubin that a caudal is less painful. Our patients who have had a caudal with a previous labour and then have a lumbar block have always been highly delighted with their experience because it is a *less* painful procedure, even though I believe that it does take longer to do. The real advantage of a caudal is that perineal analgesia is always first class. In 100 cases there was only one in whom perineal analgesia was deficient. The great advantage of a caudal is that it can be done very quickly but you must select your patients from those in whom the bony landmarks are easily palpable.

Dr Carrie (Oxford): I find myself in the position of coming to the support of the obstetricians because caudals seem to be faring worst in this discussion. In fact many caudals are still done in Oxford (500–600 per year), but they are done by the obstetricians, who are very keen on them. My own inclination as an anaesthetist is towards the lumbar route because of its precision and its proximity to the segments subserving uterine pain. But there is no doubt that the obstetricians do the caudals extremely well. I have worked with them and have been impressed by their expertise, by the efficacy of the method and their lack of complications. Their figures compare favourably with most reported series of lumbar epidurals. There has been failure to obtain satisfactory analgesia (including failure to locate the sacral hiatus) of only 4 to 5 per cent in expert hands and 11 per cent overall: there has been no significant sepsis and no marked hypotension unrelieved by turning the patient on to her side; the frequency of dural tap is 0·2%.

Another important aspect of the technique whereby the caudals are performed by the obstetricians is that this might be the answer to the demand for better obstetric analgesia in this country. Most people are agreed that epidural analgesia, be it lumbar or sacral, is the most effective method of obstetric pain relief. The great difficulty is to provide a service on a national scale. There is a more plentiful supply of obstetricians than of obstetric anaesthetists in Britain's labour wards, so a caudal service by the obstetricians is much more likely to be available to a larger number of patients. Except by greatly increasing the number of obstetric anaesthetic sessions or by teaching the obstetricians how to do lumbar epidurals this seems the only way to provide a nation-wide obstetric analgesic service.

Dr Young (Manchester): The newly set up epidural service at the United Manchester Hospitals provides for the blocks being given both by obstetricians as well as anaesthetists. The decision was made because of the relative shortage of anaesthetists and the conviction that experience in pain-relieving blocks should be part of the obstetricians' training.

Our obstetricians opted for the caudal route as being more suited to the non-specialist. It has the further advantage that all items of equipment are available as disposables except the Millipore filters and the ampoules of bupivacaine which are sterilised in individual screw-capped bottles; the filters and the bottles are returned to be used again. The use of disposable items means that the block can always be attempted on an ad hoc basis and that unexpected demands can never exhaust the supply of sterilised drums of equipment. This constant availability has already encouraged the re-introduction of spinal anaesthesia in my practice, and might be expected to do the same for epidural analgesia.

Where the caudal canal cannot be entered, the help of the anaesthetist on duty is invoked; he attempts the lumbar route. Since the lumbar epidural needle is too expensive to be regarded as disposable, the equipment is prepared together in a drum.

Dr Armstrong (Belfast): I feel that it is worth emphasising the usefulness of the caudal block in cases where conventional analgesia has failed. Under these circumstances one is faced with a restless, disturbed patient who is incapable of co-operation, thus rendering a lumbar epidural block technically impossible.

A caudal block can often be performed in these conditions, and if a 19-gauge 2 inch disposable needle is used in conjunction with a disposable syringe, the chances of a dural puncture must be remote. A single shot injection of bupivacaine usually gives sufficient duration of analgesia to ensure the completion of labour in comparative comfort.

Dr Massey Dawkins (London): I would like to take issue with Dr Rubin on the subject of dural puncture. My friend, James Cyriax of St Thomas's Hospital has done over 10,000 sacral injections for relief of low back pain and he does admit to a dural puncture rate of $1\frac{1}{2}\%$. I think that the picture is not quite as rosy as Dr Rubin paints.

"Why are Epidurals not more widely practised?"

Dr T R Steen (Bristol): 'There is one class of person to whom one speaks with difficulty, and another to whom one speaks in vain.' So wrote T S Eliot[1] at his most pontifical, and the idea may be relevant in this context. With difficulty one speaks to many obstetricians and midwives. Rightly they regard the avoidance and alleviation of pain in labour as an important part of obstetric care, and they achieve broadly satisfactory and extremely safe results with the centrally-acting analgesics with which they are familiar. Major forms of regional analgesic block imply a different approach, possibly necessitating modifications in obstetric management, and may seem incompatible with the attitudes inherent in the idea of 'natural childbirth'. Further, the involvement of an extra doctor in what should be a private occasion for the mother is better avoided unless really necessary. The unpredictable nature of obstetric work, with a high frequency of things happening at very inconvenient times constitutes another reason for obstetricians being reluctant to seek the help of their anaesthetist colleagues.

Such factors account for the slowness, which many of us have personally experienced, with which epidurals may be exploited in the obstetric department even of a hospital where they have been regularly used in surgical cases for very many years. In the wake of the publicity that followed the World Congress in 1968, I personally offered, in effect, 'epidural on demand' to the obstetricians in my hospital, where about 90 babies are born every week. A flood of requests, for which new staffing arrangements would be necessary, was anticipated; but, though results have been gratifying and there have been no complications of any consequence or severity, only about 2 epidurals per week have actually been done. An obstetric colleague explains the low demand as due to solicitude for my coronaries, and perhaps I should be grateful!

Nevertheless once they have witnessed the impressive results of the method, most obstetricians will wish to have it available, at least on special indication: surely the transformation which is regularly effected by an epidural in painful labour is one of the most beautiful things in the whole of medicine.

While a few obstetricians, with special enthusiasm and talents, may learn and practise epidural analgesia themselves, the provision of this form of pain relief will generally, and properly, fall to anaesthetists.

Turning then to anaesthetists—I am speaking now to a highly selected audience—it is because of recent trends in the specialty that one fears that to many anaesthetists one may speak in vain. A Victorian novelist complained that religion in his time had so narrowed down to a contemplation of Sin as to constitute an offence to all respectable people. By the same token, some prominent anaesthetists advise that the methods of 'Flicking the Fluotec' or 'Paralyse and Puff' are so effective, easy, safe and universally applicable, that routine anaesthesia has become too narrow a subject to merit the attention of qualified doctors, and ought to be delegated to non-medical personnel, while anaesthetists could devote much of their time to Intensive Care and so regain clinical interest in their work.[2] Other authorities challenge this sanguine view of the state of the specialty. Thus, Professor Mushin[3], in 1967, reviewing 'Clinical Anaesthesia Conferences'[4] wrote 'Its contents will give a jolt to anyone who still believes that anaesthesia is either easy or inevitably safe'. In 1970, Dr Langton Hewer,[5] touching on a subject which concerns obstetric anaesthetists very closely, asked 'What are we to make of the recent spate of reports[6][7] concerning awareness during anaesthesia and unpleasant recall after it? When these incidents excite public notice, the reaction of patients will be "if you cannot even keep us unconscious, anaesthesia must be in a pretty bad way"; and there would be good grounds for the complaint.'

Whatever the outcome of that debate, the fact remains that for some time one has often met anaesthetists well advanced in their training whose repertoire is extremely meagre and whose manual skills are limited to putting a needle in a vein or a tube in a trachea; even their bag-squeezing is done by machine. They cannot perform a lumbar puncture, still less an epidural, with much confidence.

The point that needs stressing is that puncture of the epidural space is not entirely easy, and one ought not to attempt to learn it on obstetric patients, probably restless and unco-operative, for whom the method is most likely to be requested in a hospital embarking on it for the first time. Rather should confidence and skill first be acquired in the quietness of routine lists in general operating theatres. Luckily there are hospitals where regional techniques are regularly practised and may therefore be taught and learned. I believe that, quite apart from any application to obstetrics, this policy is wise. But this is no time to argue that case. Suffice it to say that until this view is more widely accepted and acted upon, then plain unfamiliarity with regional analgesic techniques will continue, and properly continue, to constitute the main reason for their non-application.

Nobody denies that anaesthetists have special knowledge and skills which can be valuably deployed outside the narrow confines of the operating theatre. By an historical accident—namely the coincidence of the early post-war poliomyelitis epidemics with the introduction of muscle-relaxants into clinical anaesthesia—anaesthetists have been drawn into Intensive Care. Perhaps this has been inevitable, perhaps it has even been right, but one may question whether it is entirely logical. Certainly such work is not so clearly a logical extension of the anaesthetist's distinctive primary function as is this wonderful technique of pain relief in labour.

REFERENCES

1. Eliot T S (1939). *The Idea of a Christian Society*, p.14 Faber and Faber, London

2. Bourne J G (1970). *Anaesthetics: Time to Delegate?* Lancet, 1, 38

3. Mushin W W (1967). *Review of Clinical Anesthesia Conferences.* Brit. J Anaesth. 39, 793

4. Mark Lester C (1967). *Clinical Anesthesia Conferences.* J and A Churchill, London

5. Hewer C Langton (1970). *Thoughts on Modern Anaesthesia.* p.viii J and A Churchill, London

6. Wilson J and Turner D J (1969). *Awareness during Caesarean Section under General Anaesthesia.* Brit. med. J. **1**, 281

7. Crawford J S, Harley N F, Bland E P and Shah J L. (1969) *Awareness during Anaesthesia.* Brit. med. J. **1**, 508

Dr Michael Rosen (Cardiff): Although I have not widely practised lumbar epidurals for labour—my experience was quite a while ago in the United States with caudal analgesia—it seems that most people in this room believe that the lumbar route is the most successful way of managing an epidural block. It is quite clear to me, from hearing the papers today, that a high degree of skill is required to do this successfully and relatively safely. Skill is needed for administration; to set up the organisation, for preparing the equipment, for deciding what methods of asepsis shall be used and seeing that it is carried out with the proper degree of safety. There is skill in the management of the patient—that requires experience and knowledge—and there have been many problems described today which have not been answered yet. Then there is technical skill and complication rates are clearly related to it. We know that in training doctors there will be a price to pay in terms of complications which some of us may find more or less acceptable. Then I think that we have to be quite clear that although epidural analgesia is the most successful form of pain relief in obstetrics, is it not absolutely guaranteed to succeed. I would like to congratulate Dr Crawford on his very honest paper. He produced results which showed that 75% multigravida and 84% primigravida were fully satisfied, but about 25% and 16% respectively, were not. They felt some pain or discomfort in labour. So it is not total relief of pain for every patient. Then we would have to subtract a figure for the number of blocks which were tried unsuccessfully. Every series reports some failures. Gunther and Bauman[1] have quoted, in their series of caudals, some 11% which were ineffective and 9% which were excluded for other obstetric causes.

We have to consider this very successful method in two situations. Firstly, those with inco-ordinate uterine action, and also those having a very painful labour which cannot be relieved by other means. All of us would agree that these are good indications and the means should be available to help the patient. Then secondly, there are others who have presented today the use of epidurals in which the relief of pain in labour is the only indication, however mild it may be. Now we know and we have heard today, that a small percentage of patients do not feel *any* pain in labour. I have observed myself that, following the insertion of a caudal catheter, everything goes very nicely without the injection of any local anaesthetic. The patient just will not admit that she has any pain. In addition, we have to compare epidural block with conventional techniques—the use of narcotics and inhalational methods which claim 20 to 35% 'complete' pain relief, according to the mothers' opinions, and up to 90% 'complete' or 'considerable' pain relief as long as a doctor administers the analgesia. Now these are very good figures if they could be sustained. When midwives are using them, without good teaching and medical back-up the percentage of 'complete' and 'considerable' pain relief may drop as low as 70%. So part of our advance in epidurals is probably due to the presence of the doctor.

Now before we move forward into a field in which we know there is benefit, we ought to be careful that we are doing something that is necessary, that we are treating something that requires treating. As far as I know, and I stand to be corrected, there is on record no controlled clinical trial of epidural block versus other forms of analgesia in unselected patients. When that is done, then we shall be in a clearer position to see whether epidural block should be confined to patients with definite indications, which is what I believe at this point, or whether it should be freely available to every woman as a first choice.

REFERENCE

1. Gunther R E and Bauman J (1969). *Obstetrical Caudal Anesthesia: 1. A randomized study comparing 1% mepivacaine with 1% lidocaine plus epinephrine.* Anesthesiology, **31**, 5

Dr R S Atkinson (Southend-on-Sea): I have heard a great deal today, and feel rather humble in trying to add to what has already been said. Nevertheless it may be of interest to describe our experience in an ordinary district hospital where there has long been a policy of lumbar epidural block for surgical operations. Last year 750 epidurals were done for routine surgery. This is about our usual annual figure, and we all get pretty good experience, especially our junior staff. With ten members of our department, it means an average of 75 epidural blocks each. It does not work out exactly like that because the enthusiasts tend to exceed this figure and can easily top the hundred in a year, while the less keen achieve correspondingly less cases. Personally, I have usually managed between 60 and 70 a year, though in recent times I sometimes have to fight my way into doing one.

We also have about 3,500 deliveries a year in the obstetric unit. Now it is manifestly impossible for us to provide an obstetric analgesia service for these people. There is plenty of good will on the part of the obstetricians. They would like us to help more. But there is too much else to take on. You cannot run an Intensive Therapy Unit, a Cardiac Arrest service, and all the other para-anaesthetic activities that we are asked to do these days, and then take on obstetric analgesia as well. We have been reluctant to embark on more than a very limited obstetric service for various reasons. For a start the increased workload would be considerable. How many extra anaesthetists would we require to run a service to all women in labour, 24 hours a day, 7 days a week? One, two, three? And would the Regional Board agree to the increased expenditure, bearing in mind the many requests for extra staff they receive every year? We are concerned that any service to obstetric patients would be carried out by properly skilled anaesthetists, and that trainees should be closely supervised. We are aware, too, of the possibility of serious complications in a young mother. In our hospital, we have seen one patient who suffered a permanent partial paralysis of the legs following hysterectomy under epidural block. The incidence of tragic neurological complications after spinal or epidural block is exceedingly low, but we do not believe it can be entirely eliminated. When a patient requires a surgical operation, some anaesthetic risk must be accepted whether the method is general anaesthesia or epidural block. But in normal labour there is a division of opinion, and not every obstetrician or anaesthetist agrees that epidural analgesia is so superior to other methods that associated risks are acceptable.

At Southend we have had considerable experience in teaching junior staff the actual techniques of epidural block for surgical operations in theatre. We try to teach it to all who come through our department, and perhaps it is pertinent to mention some things which we think are important.

We believe it is of utmost importance always to have an indwelling needle in a vein, so that one can treat toxic effects of the local analgesic and hypotension. We also think it essential to have means of inflating the lungs with oxygen in case of respiratory failure. We do not undertake epidural block unless these two things are available. It is also important to have proper ancillary help, ability to tip the trolley and so forth.

In teaching, needles with centimetre markings are very helpful. I personally find it useful to know how far in a needle has penetrated, and one soon gets an idea of the expected depth of the epidural space in a particular build of patient.

We have also found that the 18 gauge Becton Dickinson needle is the best for teaching. The wider needle gives a better appreciation of changes in resistance to injection, so that the epidural space is more readily identified, and dural tap (we think) occurs less often. Using a syringe of air for testing, you have only to see one drop of fluid and this must be cerebrospinal fluid. A further factor which helps prevent thecal tap is rotation of the needle. The needle is advanced a few millimetres at a time, and resistance to injection of air tested in two planes at right angles to one another. Loss of resistance is quite frequently encountered 'on the turn', and this saves further advancement with the possibility of dural tap. I am pleased to say that we have an inadvertent dural puncture rate considerably lower than Dr Crawford's, and we have had several residents who have managed to complete their century by doing 100 epidurals without a dural tap. Not necessarily the first hundred, because I think it takes a good dozen or so to get the feel of the technique.

I do not think it is a good idea for beginners to use the Tuohy needle, which is difficult to use and needs a lot of force to push it in with the danger of loss of control. Nor do we use the indicators described by Dr Massey Dawkins since they are not readily available in many hospitals at the present time, whereas syringes are always in good supply. There is, however, increasing replacement of the all glass syringe by the disposable syringe. So far we have used the all glass syringe. In my experience, the disposable syringes are not so free running and tend to stick.

In teaching junior staff the following points must always be stressed. Failure is often a result of neglect of these elementary points. Firstly, get a good position of the patient with maximum flexion of the back. Secondly, take care to put in the needle at the correct angle. We teach the midline approach. Thirdly, always advance the needle *slowly* with control. Fourthly, test carefully for accidental puncture of the dura or a blood vessel. The final test is easy injection of the analgesic fluid. If this is anything but absolutely free, it is likely that the needle point is not in the epidural space.

We have explored the use of video-tape as a method of teaching. It has a place in the demonstration of nerve blocks, and we have made a tape demonstrating some different methods of locating the space.

To return to the obstetric problem, with all the other commitments of our department we are at present managing to do only about two epidural blocks a week in the labour wards, and that on special request only. Gradually this service will increase, but it will be a slow business. We are rather loath to have this launching off too fast, or to have the obstetric residents starting the technique without being properly taught the dangers and the treatment of complications.

Dr Massey Dawkins (University College Hospital): Dr Atkinson remarked that glass indicators were not readily available. The Brooks indicator can be purchased at any branch of Woolworth's for 25p. You take an ordinary household thermometer, shake out the fluid or mercury, file down the sharp end on a carborundum wheel to fit your Tuohy needle and that is all you have to do.

Mr A D Noble (Westminster Hospital): I feel very grateful that, as a young obstetrician, I am working in a unit where epidural analgesia is available to any labouring mother who needs or asks for this, surely the best, method of pain relief. As juniors, we feel that obstetric practice has radically and beneficially changed; we owe thanks to the Senior Anaesthetists and Obstetricians at Westminster whose foresight, development and planning have made this possible.

There is much agreement about the value of this method, which has been widely practised in the United States for years; so one wonders why progress here is so slow. Many reasons have been discussed by other speakers but there are others. There is prejudice, there is vested interest, there are midwives who fear that normal delivery will become obstetrician-managed, there are obstetricians who fear an increased work load of forceps deliveries and anaesthetists who are anxious regarding the increased work load. There is also the Victorian idea that the pleasure of sex must be paid for: that pain is part of labour and should be suffered. There are some who pretend to believe that the pain of labour increases the psychological ties between mother and child, or at least has some mythical ennobling effect.

I would like to tell you about some of the changes which have taken place in obstetric practice in the Westminster Hospital Group with reference to epidural analgesia (Figure 1). Initially this service was intended for patients with strictly obstetric indications. These were (a) prolonged or excessively painful labour often associated with an occipito-posterior position and unresponsive to conventional analgesics; (b) prematurity; (c) cardiac disease; (d) hypertension in labour; (e) forceps delivery. These indications were later extended to include breech and twin delivery. In later years epidural analgesia has been offered to an increasing number of mothers in normal labour. You will see from the graph that the epidural rate steadily rose as confidence was gained. Initially the forceps rate remained static because most of the patients who had an epidural would have needed forceps delivery anyway. It can be seen, however, that as epidurals were given increasingly in normal labours the forceps rate at

Figure 1

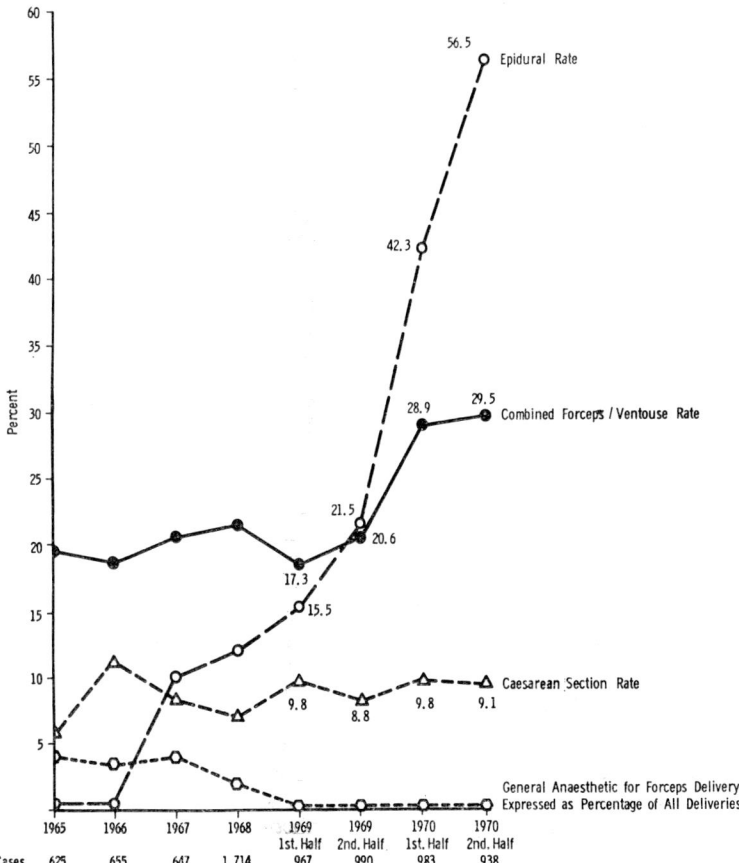

Changes in Obstetric Practice with increasing use in Epidural Analgesia.

first rose from about 20% to 30% but it now seems to have stabilised. It is noteworthy that this rise is only 10% more than the forceps rate prior to the introduction of epidural analgesia and a good deal less than many people have forecast. This problem of a rise in the forceps rate is undoubtedly a major objection to epidurals in some people's minds. In our experience the increase in work is small and is outweighed by the advantages gained because of a reduction in labour ward tension and noise.

Even with an epidural rate of about 20%, the difference in suffering between women with epidural-managed labour and that managed with conventional analgesia is glaring. The midwives, some of whom were initially prejudiced against the method, now became enthusiastic—indeed they themselves often exert pressure for a patient to be given an epidural.

The other point I would like to make is to draw attention to the bonus shown at the bottom of the graph. This shows that prior to a comprehensive epidural service, 4% of our patients required a general anaesthetic for forceps delivery. This has now been reduced to a fraction of 1%: in fact I have not performed a forceps delivery with the mother under general anaesthesia for over three years. We must remember that for the three years 1964–66 at least 50 maternal deaths in England and Wales were associated with anaesthesia[1]. Furthermore, we do not know how many other women were seriously ill with Mendelson's syndrome but survived maybe with permanent pulmonary damage. We have this bonus to set against the possible complications of epidural analgesia about which we have heard earlier today.

REFERENCE

1. Ministry of Health (1969). *Report on Confidential Enquiries into Maternal Deaths in England and Wales.* 1964-66, London, H.M.S.O.

Mr Kenneth Cooper (Worthing): Some years ago I was interested in the use of paracervical nerve block[1][2] which gave very good pain relief in about 70% of patients, but I became reluctant to continue it following reports of foetal bradycardia and still-birth after its use[3]. The work of Teramo in Scandinavia[4] showed that there was foetal acidosis when paracervical nerve block was used. So I felt that this method should be abandoned and looked round for an equally effective method of pain relief. The obvious answer lay in epidural analgesia.

Previously, I had used caudal epidural analgesia at Oxford but I had never managed to achieve the success rate of 95% that other speakers have claimed by using this route. I found that all the people with odd-shaped sacrums seemed to come my way and my results were nothing like as reliable. We decided that we would need to use the lumbar route, but the stumbling block to the setting up of the service was a shortage of anaesthetists. Anaesthetists often could not take on extra work and it was impossible to get one along at the time he was needed. It may be that at hospitals with a lot of staff an anaesthetist is appointed for obstetric anaesthesia only, but this is not the case at peripheral hospitals and it seemed that the only way to get a service going was to 'do-it-yourself'. We felt that if the epidural space approached through the caudal route was the province of obstetricians why should not the same space approached between the lumbar vertebrae also be their province? So we decided to 'do-it-ourselves'; we had enthusiasm but no special talent and naturally we sought instruction from our anaesthetic colleagues first of all. The arrangements we had were that analgesia in labour was started by pethidine injections and after the patients had received two injections of pethidine the obstetric registrar was informed. He then decided whether to continue with pethidine injections or whether to give an epidural instead. Sometimes the epidural was started earlier if we had special requests from patients, and these of course increased when they heard that the service was available.

We do the blocks in the delivery room on a firm labour bed, but after the catheter has been put in the patient is taken back to the first stage room so as to free the delivery room. We always put in a test dose first of all. A glass syringe with a freely moving plunger is ideal for detecting loss of resistance, but if used for injection through the catheter there is a disadvantage. The increased resistance to injection through the narrower catheter may cause some solution to leak back alongside the plunger and one is then uncertain as to how much has actually gone through the catheter. So we prefer to change to a plastic syringe with a tighter fit of the plunger at this point.

Top-up injections are given by the midwives, after they have had suitable instruction. The Medical Protection Society advised us that this was acceptable providing the midwives had had instruction on this. We do not put in catheters before labour has become painful.

The problems that might be expected from this are, firstly, 'midwife resistance'. This problem proved non-existent. We felt that midwives might think that we were turning normal delivery and normal cases into doctors' cases, but the converse was true. Midwives soon became enthusiastic about the method and tended to call the obstetrician to administer the epidural. The other problems you might expect would be how many mistakes beginners would make. Table 1 shows the sort of troubles experienced by 'do-it-yourself' obstetricians. In 64 lumbar epidurals we punctured the dura three times. These were given by myself and two obstetric registrars who had had very little experience with the lumbar route before. So although these things went wrong when novices tried it in 64 patients, we did relieve pain in those who would not otherwise have had adequate analgesia. These mothers were extremely grateful for the quality of pain relief which they obtained.

Table 1
Complications of Epidural Block by 'Do-it-yourself' Obstetricians

In 64 patients we:	
Punctured the dura in	3
Failed to get a satisfactory block ..	4
Cut the catheter (outside patient) ..	1
Blocked the catheter	1
Were frightened by hypotension ..	1

The advantages of the method if you do it yourself as obstetricians are, that the obstetricians being on the spot, the epidural can be done as soon as it is required. It may not be an ideal arrangement and it would probably be better if we had an obstetric anaesthetist constantly available to do it. But as we have not, it was 'do-it-yourself' or nothing. I hope that if this does not meet with too much disfavour from anaesthetists, then other obstetricians might consider doing likewise if they too are faced with the problem of either 'do-it-yourself' or going without.

REFERENCES
1. Cooper K V and Moir J C (1963). *Paracervical Block. A simple method of Pain Relief in Labour.* Brit. med. J. i, 1372
2. Cooper K, Gilroy K J and Hurry D J (1968). *Paracervical Nerve Block in Labour using Bupivacaine (Marcain).* J. Obstet. Gynaec. Brit. Cwlth. 75, 863
3. Murphy P J, Wright J D and Fitzgerald T B (1970). *Assessment of Paracervical Nerve Block Anaesthesia during Labour.* Brit. med. J. 1, 526

4. Teramo K (1969). *Foetal acid-base balance and heart rate during labour with bupivacaine paracervical block anesthesia.*
   J. Obstet. Gynaec. Brit. Cwlth. **76,** 881

OPEN DISCUSSION

The Chairman: The subject for discussion is 'Why are epidurals not more widely practised?' The possible reasons given by the five invited speakers seem to be as follows:

Dr Steen suggested that general unfamiliarity by anaesthetists with regional analgesic techniques might be responsible. This could be remedied.

Dr Rosen drew attention to the fact that epidurals are not invariably effective and perhaps we are underestimating the potential value of narcotic and inhalational methods. He is not convinced that epidural analgesia has been clearly demonstrated to be superior in efficacy and safety to the more conventional methods.

We must be grateful to Dr Atkinson and his colleagues for training so many junior anaesthetists in the technique of epidural analgesia for general surgery. Unfortunately their many other commitments preclude its frequent application in the labour wards.

Mr Noble counts himself fortunate to work in a department where epidural analgesia has been standard practice for some years, but he did mention that initially midwife prejudice had to be overcome. Now they are themselves asking for the service in individual cases.

Mr Cooper was faced with an absolute shortage of available anaesthetists which he has overcome by doing the epidurals himself.

I still feel that we may not yet have heard all the reaons why epidurals are not more widely practised.

Dr Wilson (Leeds): I have been seething with frustration throughout this discussion by the last five speakers.

I work in a large teaching hospital complex as an anaesthetist specially appointed to have charge of obstetric anaesthesia and analgesia. Interest in an epidural service is high in all ranks of the Anaesthetic Department and this is true of the junior staff in spite of the extra demands put upon them by broken nights' sleep when they have to 'top-up'. This enthusiasm is evidenced by the fact that there are three registrars with me at this meeting today.

We have always been able to staff the service apparently desired by those who appointed me eighteen months ago, but the demand for the service has been so small that juniors have had to find a large part of their epidural experience in the field of general surgery where, even there, they meet resistance to the use of this technique.

It is very difficult to understand why there is such great resistance, not only in the obstetric field, but also in the general surgical and gynaecological fields, in a particular hospital group. Many factors must be operative; in obstetrics those factors not only concern the obstetricians, but also the midwifery staff. In a recent paper one of our obstetricians stated: 'Labour pains are nature's warning of danger to the mother and baby. Painless labour can be as dangerous as a silent coronary'. He continues by stating the need for better pain control in labour and concludes: 'This technique (intravenous pethidine self-infused by the patient until pain is relieved) carries the prospect of bringing narcotic analgesia up to the level of efficacy of conduction blockade.'[1] I feel that this statement infers the great danger of painless rupture of the uterus in association with epidural analgesia, possibly in the presence of an old Caesarean section scar. It also illustrates a very clear awareness of the efficiency of epidural blockade in obstetric analgesia and this admission is of great importance to us. With regard to the question of Caesarean scar rupture and loss of 'warning pain', this is put in a different perspective by the recent article by Case et al[2] in which they pointed out the relative infrequency of pain as a guide to scar rupture.

Within my first eighteen months here it became evident from the attitude of some of my obstetric colleagues that I had little right of clinical access to the patients in the labour ward. I feel that this is one of the main factors in preventing the more widespread use of epidural analgesia. In an area where the technique has been so little practised, it will become popular only by 'patient demand' when the news of its efficacy is disseminated by the patients who have received it. Within the very recent past there has been a slight change in the attitude of two of my obstetric colleagues and I now find that I am a permitted, if not a welcome, initiator of occasional epidural blocks.

What other factors influence this attitude, not only here but in other schools? One factor may be the relative infrequency of the visits of senior obstetricians to the labour wards and therefore their absence during long, distressing labours. Overworked and relatively junior obstetric staff often order analgesia by telephone. Indeed, on these occasions the patients do obtain an element of pain relief but generally at the cost of some degree of confusion and even of impaired consciousness. As we all know, in some cases this 'narcosis' is associated with severe neonatal depression.

A further difficulty is communication of information about the technique and its demand for closer obstetric observation both by midwives and doctors. This I have personally found difficult in that, despite my appointment as obstetric anaesthetist, I do not conduct any of the formal teaching of midwives in training or those who have already been trained. This is certainly a problem associated with our own anaesthetic discipline and in no way the fault of our obstetric colleagues.

I commented on the need for closer obstetric observation required of epidural cases, and this could in theory put a greater strain on the already overworked junior obstetric staff. It takes a long time to convince them both by theory and practice that in the long run their work load may be reduced, for example, by reduction in the number of Caesarean sections carried out for maternal distress.

Resistance from midwives I have encountered, but this is natural with any new technique which virtually revolutionises the labour ward practice. On the whole resistance has not been sustained and certainly has never been antagonistic. Indeed, I have found that the midwives have put themselves out to try and understand the method, its uses and why it should be used.

I hope that the tide is turning with us now, but I can still see problems ahead and perhaps some of the obstetricians present could help with advice.

REFERENCES

1. Scott J S (1970). *Obstetric Analgesia, A consideration of labour pain and a patient-controlled technique for its relief with Meperidine.* Amer. J. Obstet. Gynec. **106**, 959

2. Case B D, Corcoran R, Jeffcoate N and Randle G H. (1971). *Caesarean Section and its place in Modern Obstetric Practice.* J. Obstet. Gynec. Brit. Cwlth. **78**, 203

Dr Burn (Southampton): At Southampton there are approximately 3,000 women delivered annually in the main obstetric unit; of these about 130 (under 5%) are given epidural analgesia in labour, despite the provision of a 24-hour 'epidural' service. In order to discover why epidurals are not employed more frequently, a small survey was recently conducted. It involved sending questionnaires to all the obstetricians and anaesthetists (senior and junior) and to all midwifery sisters; and a random sample of patients, some of whom had received epidural analgesia during labour and some of whom had not, were interviewed personally. The numbers involved (35 medical staff, 25 midwives and 30 patients) were too small to provide valid statistics, although there was fairly good uniformity of opinion on specific questions. Unfortunately the answers did not reflect what is practised, and although lip service is paid to the value of epidurals, the above figures speak for themselves.

From the survey and from personal experience in the unit, there emerge a host of reasons why epidurals are not more widely used; but basically these are summarised by: complacency, ignorance, prejudice and inertia. More specifically the reasons can be enumerated under the following headings:

Patients: Many patients are ignorant of the existence and benefits of epidural analgesia, and hence there is a lack of patient demand. Of those who have heard about epidurals, some were concerned about the possible risks of complications ('paralysis') to themselves, or of the adverse effect it might have on the foetus. A small number felt strongly that they did not want to miss the physical sensation associated with birth, even if this entails pain. These apart, all who received epidurals were delighted and wanted to have one 'next time'; while over half who did not have an epidural claimed that they did not get good pain relief in their labour.

Midwives: Nearly all midwives considered pain in labour was inevitable and acceptable, and that the conventional methods of relief were quite adequate. They are unaware of the substantial advantages—apart from analgesia—that derive from the use of epidurals, namely improved placental circulation, reduction of blood pressure in pre-eclamptic toxaemia, the absence of foetal respiratory depression or risk of maternal inhalation of vomitus, the reduced blood loss in the third stage, and—as we have heard today—the benefit to maternal and foetal acid-base equilibrium. They consider the risks and complications outweigh any benefit in pain relief, except in selected cases where there is an obstetric indication for an epidural. Trained midwives, they feel, would lose some of their responsibility, and the pupil midwives would find it difficult to obtain sufficient experience of normal deliveries. Many thought that the management of a patient having an epidural entailed closer supervision, and therefore more work for the nursing staff. The incursion of the anaesthetists into this field, except in special cases, is not altogether appreciated and midwives prefer to manage pain relief in labour independently. The suggestion that all primiparous women should be offered an epidural was completely rejected.

Obstetricians: From the lack of requests for epidural analgesia one can only presume, contrary to the replies obtained in the survey, that there is satisfaction with the conventional methods of analgesia in labour, and the advantages and superiority of epidural analgesia are not conceded. Concern over the risks of complications seems to be directly proportional to the degree of ignorance about the actual complications and their (usually simple) treatment. Again, this leads to the request for epidurals being made only on special grounds rather than as a routine form of pain relief. It is feared too that the work load on the midwives and junior obstetric staff would be excessive from the wider use of epidurals. Perhaps also, as with the midwives, assistance involving dependence upon non-obstetric staff, is not altogether welcomed unless it is necessary to resolve a particular problem.

Anaesthetists: There is unfortunately a numerical lack of anaesthetists who either can, or are willing to do obstetric epidurals. To justify this inertia and lack of interest, it is claimed that conventional methods are quite adequate; though the most cursory visit to any obstetric unit should convince anyone that—as practised generally—such methods are far from perfect. It is felt too that the risks and complications outweigh any advantages, except where epidurals are specially indicated; but as the experience of 'non-epidural' anaesthetists in this field is limited (or non-existent) these fears are based more on ignorance than fact. No doubt they have the tag '*primum non nocere*' uppermost in their minds, assuming that by doing nothing to relieve pain they can do no harm; ignoring the fact that 'conventional' methods themselves carry definite risks and complications also. They do not feel that every primiparous woman should be offered an epidural; but cite the occasional errors (usually dural puncture) made by inexperienced anaesthetists (who should anyway learn the technique in theatre first) as an argument against this sort of service being advocated at all. The more honest merely say it is 'too demanding' a technique.

Epidurals, if properly practised, provide obstetric analgesia second to none in efficacy, and also have many other important advantages. It may require some effort on the part of the anaesthetists and obstetricians, and it may (possibly rightly) relieve midwives of some responsibility; but the appreciation of women, who have enjoyed the benefit of it, is eloquent testimony to its worth. The reasons that it is not practised more widely are largely invalid, and when complacency, ignorance, prejudice and inertia can be removed, then epidurals will be used far more frequently to the benefit of women in labour. The prime responsibility lies with anaesthetists to interest themselves in the problem and, by their efforts, convince their obstetric colleagues and midwives of the undoubted value of the technique.

Dr Rosen (Cardiff): Perhaps I am in a minority, but I am still not absolutely satisfied as to what are the general risks of serious complications with epidurals. On the one hand, we hear of series by some who never have any troubles. They have had dural punctures but apparently no

113

complications from them. The two dural punctures with Tuohy needles that I have seen both got nerve pareses which ultimately recovered in about ten to fourteen days. It seems unlikely that this only happens in Cardiff. The patients recovered, it is true, but it was unpleasant at the time and one of the husbands asked many awkward questions. Then there is the incidence of permanent nerve pareses. Dr Massey Dawkins has told us that it is 0·02%. That is not very much, but we do approximately 5,000 deliveries a year in Cardiff, and therefore we would have one every year! I would like those who have a done a lot of epidurals as at the Westminster Hospital, who do 80% of their cases in this way, to tell us whether they have had any serious complications; and perhaps Dr Selwyn Crawford could say specifically what he has seen in the vast numbers he met when he was in the United States. If we could be reassured about this in tens of thousands of patients then I think many would feel easier about going forward. But until we do I think that this is one of the major factors which make us all cautious about advancing the use of this technique on a very widespread scale.

Dr J Selwyn Crawford (Birmingham): I can quote two sets of experiences. In Birmingham we have now done more than 1,200 lumbar epidurals and have had no serious complications, that is if you define headache following a dural puncture as not being 'serious' in terms of long-term patient welfare. We have had one patient who had a patch of loss of sensation on the outer aspect of one thigh for up to three weeks post-partum. This had cleared by the time she came for the post-natal visit 6 weeks after delivery. That is the only neurological complication or any other of note which we have met in the 1,200.

With regard to what happens on the other side of the Atlantic, I think that there exists a fairly glib impression that lumbar epidurals are widely practised in the United States and Canada. They are not given to anything like that extent. In American obstetric practice, the majority of regional blocks are saddle blocks, just for the second stage and for the delivery. They define that as being relief of pain in labour ignoring the 8 or 12 hours of pain that has gone before. The incidence of caudal blocks is much higher than that of lumbar epidurals. I would suggest that within the next 5 or 10 years in this country we will have had nationally much more experience of lumbar epidural block in labour than in the United States.

Dr Hargrove (Westminster Hospital): As you know, we offer epidural analgesia to all mothers in labour and have given approximately 1,200 blocks in the last 12 months. To my knowledge, in that time, we have had about 15 dural taps and two of these have resulted in, what I would consider to be, complications.

In the first patient the headache lasted 14 days with a lot of neck stiffness, which cleared completely at the end of the fortnight. The other patient had a headache, neck stiffness and a 6th nerve palsy. The palsy lasted 8 weeks, but also cleared up completely. This was in an ex-Westminster Hospital midwife who was the wife of a dental surgeon, so she was obviously a first class candidate for something to go wrong! I also feel that neither patient was adequately managed following their dural tap, since the first patient was not immediately put on complete bed rest, and the second patient was found to have had 5 days' treatment with a diuretic in order to suppress lactation. I am sure that this aggravated her symptoms.

Dr Felicity Reynolds (St Thomas's Hospital, London): I find it difficult to understand why obstetricians continue to resist the use of epidural analgesia while continuing to accept respiratory depression of babies born to mothers who have received very large doses of pethidine. The ready passage of pethidine across the placenta is well recognised and I would be very willing to measure neonatal pethidine levels to add to the armoury of argument of those who wish to battle for the wider use of epidural analgesia.

Summing Up

The Chairman: The time has come for your Chairman to shed his mantle of impartiality, reveal himself as highly biased, and sum up this debate. Many and various are the reasons why epidurals are not widely practised. Those who may have been inspired by today's proceedings to start an epidural service in their own hospitals will find their paths beset by obstacles, most of them, I hope, removable. The keys to success are the firm desire of the obstetricians to see the service established and the determination of their anaesthetists to get it going. The midwives, so often represented as the chief opponents of change, can be converted to enthusiastic allies by instruction, re-assurance and seeing for themselves the benefits of properly managed epidural analgesia. A prophet is not without honour save in his own country; a visitation by a prophet from another centre to give a lecture and a demonstration could be the spark to enkindle local interest.

One must respect the views of those who have misgivings about the more frequent use of epidural analgesia, but even they admit that it is indicated in 'selected' cases. It is agreed that safety and skill can only be achieved by constant practice. Surely a certain number of epidurals must be done regularly in an obstetric department to ensure that they can be done safely and skilfully when really 'necessary' by the anaesthetist who happens to be on duty at the time.

We must sympathise with those who find themselves too short of staff to provide a frequent service. Paradoxically I have found that the more frequently epidurals are given the easier it is to provide a competent service in the individual case. Every obstetric department has to be covered for general anaesthesia. Setting up an epidural should be far less consuming of time and effort than giving a general anaesthetic. If this can be achieved then the service can be assimilated with the other duties of the on-call anaesthetist with the bonus that it avoids the need to call him for an operative vaginal delivery.

What happens in centres where epidurals are simply not available? Do conventional analgesic methods really compare favourably with a competent epidural service in efficacy, reliability and acceptability to the patient? Can we continue to tolerate the situation in which epidural analgesia is accepted and sought after in private practice while anaesthetists beg to be allowed to apply the technique in the hospitals of the National Health Service?

INDEX